THE TEACCH APPROACH TO AUTISM SPECTRUM DISORDERS

THE TEACCH APPROACH TO AUTISM SPECTRUM DISORDERS

Gary B. Mesibov

University of North Carolina
Chapel Hill, NC

Victoria Shea

University of North Carolina
Chapel Hill, NC

and

Eric Schopler

University of North Carolina
Chapel Hill, NC

with

Lynn Adams	Elif Merkler
Sloane Burgess	Matt Mosconi
S. Michael Chapman	Christine Tanner
Mary E. Van Bourgondien	

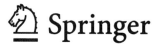 Springer

The TEACCH approach to autism spectrum disorders / Gary B. Mesibov,
Victoria Shea, Eric Schopler.
 p. ; cm.
Includes bibliographical references and index.
ISBN 0-306-48646-6 (hardbound)
1. Autism. I. Mesibov, Gary B. II. Shea, Victoria. III. Schopler, Eric.
[DNLM: 1. Autistic Disorder—rehabilitation. 2. Education, Special—methods.
3. Professional-Family Relations. WM 203.5 T2528 2004]
RC553.A88T43 2004
618.92′85882—dc21

2004051533

ISBN 0-306-48647-4

Springer Science+Business Media, Inc.
233 Spring Street, New York, New York 10013

springeronline.com

10 9 8 7 6 5 4 3 2

A C.I.P. record for this book is available from the Library of Congress.

Preface

For over 30 years, Treatment and Education of Autistic and related Communication handicapped Children (TEACCH) has been an innovator in developing and implementing a state-wide system for assisting and supporting people with autism spectrum disorders and their families in North Carolina. The TEACCH program has both served the citizens of North Carolina and been a model for services throughout the country and all over the world. TEACCH has developed a conceptual model for understanding autism spectrum disorders (called the Culture of Autism) that has facilitated comprehension of autism spectrum disorders by parents and professionals. This understanding, in turn, has yielded a set of intervention strategies (called Structured Teaching) that provide an organizing foundation for classrooms, homes, and community-based services throughout the world.

The purpose of this book is to describe the TEACCH program and explain its many facets that reflect the conceptual model, based on the notion that autism is a neuropsychological disorder and that intervention strategies should be closely linked to empirical findings about neuropsychological functioning in autism.

The first chapter, which was written by Eric Schopler, the co-founder of TEACCH, traces the history of the TEACCH program. Chapter 2, written by Gary Mesibov, the current Director of TEACCH, delineates the core values that those working in the organization share and espouse. Chapters 3 and 4 introduce the TEACCH concept of the Culture of Autism and describe the Structured Teaching approach, and Chapter 5 explains the relationship of the TEACCH approach to other theoretical models. Chapters 6 and 7 cover the empirical literature and describe the strategies TEACCH has developed for teaching communication and social skills that people with ASD need to be successful in our society. Elif Merkler and Matt Mosconi made major contributions to the chapter on social skills.

Chapters 8 and 9 describe the research literature about parents of individuals with autism, and review TEACCH's multi-faceted work with parents, including ways that TEACCH professionals communicate with them about their youngster's autism and its implications. Chapters 10 and 11 discuss the application of TEACCH principles to the specialized populations of preschool children and adults with autism, respectively. Christie Tanner and Sloane Burgess took the lead in writing the preschool chapter, and the adult chapter was written by Mary Beth Van Bourgondien and Mike Chapman. Finally, Chapter 12, written by Lynn Adams, addresses the issue of training professionals to understand the TEACCH approach.

Although the authors who have taken the responsibility for organizing and writing the various sections are those listed on the book cover, this book is, in reality, the work of a much larger number of people over many years. There are too many of them to acknowledge individually but their hard work, support, and commitment are the heart of what the TEACCH program has become. Special thanks are also offered to our publishers, Kluwer Academic/Plenum Publishers, for their patience and support of this project and especially our Editor, Mariclaire Clouiter. Our wonderful secretarial staff including Joan Berry and Jill Cagle provided typing and all of the administrative support in their usual efficient and gracious fashion. Of course the major source of inspiration for this book is the people with ASD themselves and their courageous families, who teach us every day about autism and how people can face a difficult challenge with great courage, persistence, and class. They elevate all of us who are privileged to know and work with them.

Contents

THE TEACCH APPROACH TO AUTISM SPECTRUM DISORDERS

CHAPTER 1

The Origins and History of the TEACCH Program

INTRODUCTION

The TEACCH Program as it exists at the time of this publication has served thousands of individuals and families involved with the challenges and problems of the autism spectrum. It now employs hundreds of staff with multi-disciplinary training. The program's mission, priorities, services, and practices are the product of the thoughtful, dedicated work and contributions of many faculty and staff. This chapter is intended to trace the motivating factors shaping the development and history of the program.

My interest in autism first took shape while I (Eric Schopler) was in graduate school at the University of Chicago when a psychology professor by the name of Bruno Bettelheim shared his excitement about the University Orthogenic School he had taken over. He said that he was solving the puzzle of the 'mental illness' of autism by removing affected children from their parents and keeping them as long as possible at his residential school. He taught the counselors at the school that emotionally cold parents had produced the autistic features in their children through unconscious feelings of hostility and rejection. These parents were, he said, like concentration camp guards, and the children were the victims, just as he himself had been a concentration camp victim in Nazi Germany.

During the years of my graduate studies I was fortunate to have worked at an outpatient clinic serving families of children with autism or primary disorders of childhood, as they were sometimes referred to at that time. They were also referred to as psychotic, symbiotic psychosis, atypical, schizophrenic, and other labels, with no agreement among professionals as to how these labels distinguished children. Based on my work there I came to believe that Bettelheim's extreme views about autism were misguided and likely to have negative consequences for children, families, and any others falling under his influence. In fact, Bettelheim became a 'negative role model' for me (Schopler, 1993) who made me recognize the need for replacing the dominant misleading psycho-analytic theories about autism with empirical research, because this would be necessary in order to develop a viable service program. The following studies, mostly conducted while developing the TEACCH Program, seemed pivotal to shaping program priorities.

PIVOTAL STUDIES FOR DEVELOPING TEACCH

My first study was my doctoral dissertation (Schopler, 1966) which was de-signed to show that autism was not an emotional illness caused by unconscious parental errors in child rearing, but, instead, that autism and related develop-mental disorders were primarily impaired ways of experiencing the world and understanding that experience. This included impaired and unusual sensory processes, unusual ways of thinking and understanding, restricted social inter-actions, impaired communication, and restricted interests.

The first step in my research was the hardest to demonstrate: that autism was not primarily a disorder of emotions, but a disorder of processing sensory information affecting smell, taste, hearing, vision, and pain sensation (Schopler, 1965). Before going to graduate school I had observed that many children with autism tended to smell and touch things but were frequently inattentive to audi-tory or visual information. In my dissertation study, we used three comparison groups: children who were developing normally, children with mental retarda-tion, and children with autism. I wanted to study their preference for visual or tactile forms of exploration. The children were provided with four objects to be compared by either visual or tactile properties. The objects included a visual display of stuffed animals compared to the same animals secured for only tactile exploration, blocks with variations in texture but of the same color compared with multicolored blocks with no texture differences, and jig saw puzzles to be assembled according to the properties of color and form versus puzzles matched only by shape. The length of exploratory time spent on each situation was com-pared for all groups. I found that in the typically-developing group, the younger children spent more time on tactile and less time on visual processes than the older children. On the tasks as a whole, the children with mental retardation did not differ from the typical children in amount of time spent on visual processes. But the autistic group spent less time on visual processes than on tactile ones compared to either of the other groups.

A little while later we followed up my doctoral study with a factor analysis (Reichler & Schopler, 1971) of scores on the Childhood Autism Rating Scale (CARS; Schopler, Reichler, Devillis, & Daly, 1980; Schopler, Reichler, & Renner, 1988) to see whether children's perceptual peculiarities were related to their problems with human and social relationships—problems now recognized as a central feature of autism. The analysis revealed three factors, including a measure of human relatedness and of social perceptual functions. A further regression analysis showed that much of the variance in human relatedness was accounted for by the variation in the perceptual scores. This analysis supported our informal observations that:

1. Much of the social impairment in autism may be due to perceptual peculiarities.
2. Much inappropriate maternal behavior—or what may appear as inappropriate—is in response to such peculiarities, rather than being the cause of them.
3. Both could be modified and improved with education.

From these two formal studies we concluded that we were on the right track in looking to education as the main venue for change and improvement.

We realized, however, that our formal studies comparing the use of visual and tactile modalities did not say anything about the use of other perceptual systems. My doctoral research only compared preferences for the distance receptor system of vision versus the near receptor system of touch, but other sensory and cognitive systems were of course also involved in daily living. Although a researcher could easily spend an entire career on any of these, we were concerned with helping a highly misunderstood and underserved group via education. So the question for us became, were there any problems of learning and thinking that were peculiar to autism? Relying on informal observation, we concluded that a majority of people in the autism spectrum learned much better using their visual modality than their auditory modality. This insight has been built into our structured learning methods since then, and has had cross-cultural replication internationally (Schopler and Mesibov, 2000).

STUDIES OF EDUCATIONAL PRACTICES

Back in 1970, in order to apply our observations about special learning problems in autism we had to evaluate and figure out how to modify the prevailing practice in U.S. special education that considered autism to be an emotional illness and therefore taught children in classrooms for the emotionally disturbed.

This educational practice was based on the Freudian theory suggesting that the primary solution to the problem of emotionally disturbed children was to remove the emotional pressures due to excessive parental expectations by giving the children a maximum amount of freedom in how they wished to use their educational experience. Often as not, this produced a very chaotic environment for 'learning.'

We decided to make a formal study of these ideas by rotating a group of children with autism from structured to unstructured sessions over two repeated two-week cycles (Schopler, Brehm, Kinsbourne, & Reichler, 1971). In the structured session, the adult decided on the materials to be used, the length of time, and how to use them. In the unstructured session, the child selected the material, how long, and in what manner to work with it. Two independent raters rated the children's behavior for attention span, appropriate communication, and behavioral problems. We found that the children responded better to structured than unstructured conditions, and that children with lower developmental functions became more disorganized the less structure they had.

Because of the variability in children's level of disability, and the apparent uniqueness of their specific learning problems, we concluded that special diagnostic instruments for autism would be needed. We designed the CARS in an effort to take the diagnostic confusion resulting from the many differing diagnostic labels cited above, and interpreted by the esoteric criteria of subjective theory, and to replace it with ratings of observable behaviors, as made by a public rating scale. It was evident that these psychometrically reliable and valid ratings of shared characteristics, to be grouped in a diagnostic category, were not sufficient for designing an optimum educational program. In addition, a developmental assessment would be needed for each child, to determine the level of structure and the individual variations in different functions of learning.

The diagnostic grouping would be accomplished with the Childhood Autism Rating Scale (CARS; Schopler et al., 1988), a diagnostic scale with established reliability and validity. The developmental assessment of each child's unique strength and weakness in learning was accomplished with the creation of the Psychoeducational Profile (PEP; Schopler and Reichler, 1979), its subsequent revision (PEP-R; Schopler, Reichler, Bashford, Lansing, and Marcus, 1990), and now the third revision (PEP-3; Schopler, Lansing, and Marcus, in press). This type of assessment was also extended for older individuals via the Adolescent and Adult Psychoeducational Profile (AAPEP; Mesibov, Schopler, Schaffer, and Landrus, 1988), now revised to the TEACCH Transition Assessment Profile (TTAP; Mesibov, Schopler, Thomas, Chapman, and Denzler, in press).

STUDIES OF PARENTS

Another pivotal aspect of our early research pertained to the understanding of parents—an issue raised so pointedly by Bettelheim at the University of Chicago. His deeply hostile attitude towards mothers was recently documented in Pollak's (1997) scholarly monograph in which he reported the expression of negative parental attitudes in Bettelheim's school practices and policies. Regular school visits by parents were not allowed, and an abstract stone sculpture of a large breasted female figure was placed in the play yard so the children could learn through play on the stone statue, that their mother had a heart cold as stone. His attitude was also revealed in the metaphor he wrote: "When one is forced to drink black milk from dawn to dusk, whether in the death camps of Germany, or while lying in a luxurious crib, but there subjected to the unconscious death wishes of what may be a conscientious mother,—in either situation, a living soul has death for a master" (Pollak, 1997, p. 143).

Bettelheim's antagonism toward mothers was somehow displaced from his own attitude towards Nazi concentration guards to the mothers of the children with autism at his school. This sort of displaced fury is called "scapegoating" and refers to blaming someone for your own frustration (Allport, 1966). I found this concept of scapegoating applicable to the prevailing mental health system attitudes toward autism at that time (Schopler, 1971).

Allport had proposed that feelings of frustration, guilt, and anxiety, among others, were catalysts for the phenomenon of scapegoating. At that time, there was no agreement about the nature of autism, its causes, its course, or optimum treatment. This confusion and lack of knowledge placed a frustrating burden on clinicians and others responsible for treating these children. Further, lack of knowledge and lack of effectiveness weighed heavily on clinicians and was often experienced as guilt and anxiety. It was much easier to blame parents than to bear the burden of this frustration and guilt. Finally, the clinician confronted with a child with autism had the burden of coping with a child who may be irritable, uncommunicative, and act as if he were alone. Since the resulting anger could not easily be expressed against the child, parents again provided a convenient substitute.

Other elements that typically lead to scapegoating were also evident in the mental health system at that time. Feelings of inferiority generated by a disorder in which the diagnosis, cause of the disorder, and treatment progress are uncertain evoke a clinician's need for self-enhancement, and the existing traces of anxiety, guilt, and desperation in parents provided a convenient handle for interpreting them as a primary cause of the child's autism. There was also an element of conformity, with pressure on new group members, specifically new clinicians, to share these beliefs. Finally, there was an aspect of tabloid thinking: rather than struggling with the questions raised by the autism disorder, it was less trouble and simpler to think in clichés or labels such as 'refrigerator mother,' 'schizophrenogenic parents,' or 'smothering mothers,' terms that had been used in the professional literature of the day. My conclusion about the scapegoating of parents was that it could best be ameliorated through empirical research, education, and professional training.

A number of influential mental health researchers had published claims that parents of severely disturbed children, including those with autism, suffered from thought disorders transmitted to their children, who would then develop autism or childhood schizophrenia. Since this seemed an extension of the scapegoating process, it was important to examine this unlikely causal explanation with formal experimental research.

In the first study (Schopler & Loftin, 1969a), we selected three groups of parents matched for their children's age. The first group had children with autism, the second group had children with mental retardation, and the third group had typically-developing children. We used the Goldstein-Scherer Object Sorting Test (OST) in which the subject is given a variety of objects and is asked to select those with any shared properties. Using this test, Lovibond (1954) had constructed categories of thought impairment whose degree could be objectively measured. Four studies had already shown that parents of children with autism demonstrated more impaired thinking than normal comparison groups and that mothers' thinking was more impaired than that of fathers.

We replicated these studies and also found that, using the OST, parents of children with autism showed more impaired thinking than the comparison group. However, on examining our data we noted that a number of the parents were in conjoint, Freudian-based therapy with their child with autism in order to 'understand' their own child-rearing 'errors.' We thought that perhaps these parents had been tested in connection with their clinic visits for therapy. It seemed quite possible that their feelings of guilt and parental failure, engendered by therapy based on Freudian theories, had produced anxiety that affected their test scores.

To examine this possibility we decided to repeat the study with three new groups of parents (Schopler & Loftin, 1969b). This time we selected a group of parents who had a child with autism and also a child who was developing normally. These parents were informed that they were invited to participate in research whose purpose was to study how parents who have a problem child are able to raise their other children successfully in getting along at school, at home, and with their friends. They were interviewed on a standard questionnaire in which they were asked about situations they were most proud of for each child. They were encouraged to tell how they reached this accomplishment and what advice they might have for other parents. After this, they were then given the Object Scoring Test with the explanation that this was not so much a test of right and wrong answers, but a test that would reveal the styles of thinking associated with successful child rearing.

With this positive test-taking situation, the mothers of children with autism scored no differently on the thought disorder task than did parents of either of the other control groups (typical children and children with mental retardation). This showed that when parents of children with autism were tested for conceptual thinking in the context of their typical child, they showed less impairment than parents tested in the context of their child with autism. The differences in thinking that had been reported between mothers and fathers also disappeared. This study clearly suggested that the thought processes of parents, especially mothers of children with autism, could become impaired or disorganized by being negatively judged or evaluated by authority figures, which suggested that some of the psychotherapy in use at that time may have produced results detrimental to the progress of both child and parents.

One of the ways in which blaming the parents had an impact on the treatment of their children was in regard to parental reports about their child's developmental problems. Professionals' mistrust of the accuracy of these reports was widespread. In light of our previous study, we designed another study (Schopler & Reichler, 1972) to test the hypothesis that if parents did not show unusual thought disorders, they should also be able to estimate the variation in developmental function so common for the autism spectrum. A group of 47 fathers and mothers, all parents of a child with autism, were asked to estimate their child's level of functioning in overall development, language, motor skills, social skills, self-sufficiency, and mental development. These estimates were then compared with those based on standard psychological testing.

As a group, these parents evaluated the variations in their child's developmental function along lines that were consistent with the standard testing. Mothers, who typically spent more time with their child than the fathers, tended to make better estimates than the fathers. (Marked disparity in developmental estimates between fathers and mothers usually indicated poor communication between them or marital discord, possibly requiring separate counseling.) Mothers with children in the mild end of the autistic spectrum were slightly more confused and less accurate in their evaluations than the mothers of children in the moderate to severe end of the spectrum. We concluded that for certain purposes, when psychological testing was not available (as in some rural districts), parents' estimates of variations in their child's developmental function could serve as a useful educational guide for developing an individualized educational program. This form was also seen a clinically helpful and has been used in TEACCH evaluations since. It has been incorporated and normed as part of PEP-3 (Schopler et al., in press).

SUMMARY OF EARLY RESEARCH

These research projects, all published in peer-reviewed professional journals, were instrumental in formulating the direction of our program and establishing the major working principles that have guided it for more than three decades. The first three pertained to the children:

1. Changing from theories of emotional causality to observable styles of perception and cognition
2. Showing the effects of perceptual styles on social relationships
3. Demonstrating educational needs for structure

The second three projects pertained to parents:

1. Showing that they were erroneously scapegoated by professionals using Freudian assumptions
2. Demonstrating that parents did not suffer from thought disorders when tested under positive conditions
3. Showing that parents were usually capable of understanding their own children's developmental levels with a significant degree of clinical accuracy

The program implications of these studies were that:

- Parents were recognized as reliable reporters of their children's problems and their history information was significant and clinically useful.
- Parents can function as co-therapists and are essential collaborators with professionals.

- Parental enthusiasm and interest is an important element in the child's improvement.
- Parent-professional collaboration facilitates important elements of service development, from program direction to the development of new services.
- Parents are essential for all advocacy functions, including legislation, political support, and the creation of greater community understanding of autism.

INITIAL YEARS OF THE TEACCH PROGRAM

During the first six years (1966–1972) of what has become the TEACCH program, I had a research grant from the National Institutes of Mental Health to investigate some of the ideas described above. I had found a young child psychiatrist in residency training at UNC, Robert Reichler, who became interested in my research on receptor processes, and I persuaded him to join me in looking at the clinical implications of my findings. We therefore took on some pilot cases and started the Child Research Project (Schopler and Reichler, 1971).

In this project, children fitting the diagnosis of autism were included, while their parents were treated as co-therapists instead of as causes of the problem. In order to carry out the co-therapy process, we decided we would observe children and parents interacting, which meant that a one-way window separating a teaching room from an observation room was needed. This one-way arrangement facilitated demonstrations of intervention techniques by therapists, and was also helpful in leading therapists to confine their recommendations to observable management techniques rather than impractical advice. Our co-therapy model also used a generalist model of intervention in which therapists alternated roles as parent consultant and child therapist. This prevented excessive identification with either the child or the parent.

One of the things we learned was that even though all the children shared the diagnosis of autism, they were really quite different from each other in behavior and cognitive style, degree of autism, learning styles, learning problems, temperament, social attachment, language, and so on. It became clear that individualized assessment was necessary. It also became clear that, in addition to studying their near-distant receptor usage, we needed to know more about each child's cognitive and behavioral issues, and more about their use of their visual and auditory senses to process information, since we had observed in the clinic a preference for visual rather than auditory processing.

SECOND PHASE OF THE TEACCH PROGRAM

In the second phase of the TEACCH program, from 1972 through 1978, we sought to convert our knowledge and research findings into social and political support. Since the NIMH grant had expired, we prepared to introduce a bill into the state legislature in order to fund continued education and research on autism. To test whether our enthusiasm for the idea of parents as co-therapists would translate to other areas of the state, we invited the lawmakers to a special breakfast get-together in order to meet our families and their very special children. This ultimately resulted in the passage of a state law mandating our program. At first there were only three regional TEACCH centers, but in later years this increased to nine centers plus our residential farm program, The Carolina Living and Learning Center (see Chapter 11, Adult Services). Children with autism were mandated by this same law to attend public school, which included funding for eleven classrooms. Now this number has expanded to almost 300 public school classrooms, staffed by teachers and assistant teachers trained in our TEACCH procedures.

During these years, we began developing the necessary formal evaluation procedures—the CARS, the PEP, and the AAPEP. We also recognized the importance to our parents and our staff of rapid access to research that would describe the latest and best intervention breakthroughs. To facilitate this, I accepted the editorship of the Journal of Autism and Childhood Schizophrenia. As we saw increasing acceptance of the understanding that autism is not really a mental illness, but rather a developmental disorder, we changed the journal's name to the Journal of Autism and Developmental Disorders (Schopler, Rutter, & Chess, 1979). We also held annual autism conferences, which later became our TEACCH Annual Conference, and edited our first collection of current research topics (with Plenum Press), which became the 13-volume series on Autism Issues. We also began what became our five-volume assessment series published by PRO-ED, which covers the individual assessment of children and adults, teaching strategies for parents and professionals, and teaching activities geared to developmental function areas used in the PEP and AAPEP. We identified preferred behavior management techniques, published subsequently (Mesibov, Schopler, & Hearsey, 1994; Schopler, 1995; Schopler, Mesibov, & Hearsey, 1995), and techniques for assessing and teaching the development of spontaneous communication (Watson, Lord, Schaffer, & Schopler, 1989). I joined the editorial board of the main NIMH mental health journals and of the Schizophrenia Bulletin, served on NIMH grant review committees, and worked on the autism subgroup of the Diagnostic and Statistical Manual of the American Psychiatric Association, taking an active part in formulating the official diagnostic criteria for autism. During this period, the TEACCH program was recognized as a cutting edge intervention for the autism spectrum by the American Psychiatric Association (Campbell, Schopler, Mesibov, & Sanchez, 1995).

Another major challenge was for us to develop active and workable collaboration with other agencies, professional organizations, and the community. I helped convert our early parent group into the first North Carolina State Advocacy Group for Autism, and was involved in the creation of the first national advocacy group, now called the Autism Society of America, becoming its first chairman of the Professional Advisory Panel.

An important collaboration was begun with the North Carolina Department of Public Instruction, including a regular liaison with the state office and a system of consultation with public school classroom teachers and assistants affiliated with TEACCH. We conducted annual intensive summer training for teachers and other school personnel, and also provided an annual Winter In-service for TEACCH-affiliated teachers and assistants. The Winter In-services were designed to fulfill two purposes. One was to find a platform for the most experienced and talented teachers and therapists in our program to identify any procedures they found to be especially effective with our children, and to present this to others in our program who might find it of help in their work. The second was to include an outside speaker who had developed a different, but related, intervention that could possibly make a new contribution to the education of children with autism and might be made compatible with our program. Such interventions have included behavioral therapy, sensory integration, music therapy, floor time therapy, and many others – all interesting, though not all equally compatible with our TEACCH approach to autism.

During this period we started our first week-long training programs for physicians, teachers, social workers, speech therapists, and all other professionals with a major concern with autism. We also worked hard towards initiating international collaboration. We had already established productive collaboration with British colleagues concerned with autism, including Michael Rutter, Lorna Wing, and their collaborators at the Maudsley Hospital in London, (Rutter & Schopler, 1978). We soon formed an international network of parents and professionals concerned with the autism spectrum, including individuals in Canada, Switzerland, Greece, Netherlands, Belgium, France, Italy, South America, Sweden, China, and Japan.

THIRD PHASE OF THE TEACCH PROGRAM

Our third phase extended roughly from 1978 through 1983. During this time, our emphasis on learning directly from children and their families took a new direction. From the very beginning, our parents had had a primary role in helping us decide the direction of our service and intervention research. By 1978, as many of the children in our original program were getting older, our parent advocacy group developed a new priority for working with adolescents and adults. Both parents and professionals recognized by then that most children with autism would not 'recover' by the time they reached adolescence, but the social service system was not set up to deal with the problems of living arrangements and vocational placement for adults with this kind of disability. Our program thus established a new mission of developing services for adolescents and adults.

I was extremely fortunate to persuade Gary Mesibov to join our program in order to spearhead this project, because of his commitment to excellence, his capacity for working collaboratively, and his commitment to effective service and social responsibility. Gary took the lead in developing our program for adult services, and later, as Director of TEACCH, he refined our summer training program to a level of excellence that continues to be praised by participants today. With him as my co-editor, we took on the 15-year project of compiling and editing a series of books on the major issues in autism that would keep our staff, our colleagues, and parents abreast of the latest issues in autism research.

During this period the Autism Society of North Carolina (ASNC), with our collaboration, developed one of the first summer camps designed for children with autism, which is now known as Camp Royall. ASNC itself continued to thrive, developing one of the strongest parent groups and providing the best mail order bookstore on autism in the United States.

CURRENT STATUS OF THE TEACCH PROGRAM

From 1984 to the present, we have developed programs for adults, including Social Skill Groups, Supported Employment, an expansion of our Winter In-Service training, and additional training in all the regional centers, and in many countries around the world (Schopler & Mesibov, 2000). The program has continued decreasing the alienating distance between individuals in the autism spectrum and the mainstream society shaped by increasingly rapid changes in technology and economic pressures. We began by replacing the existing gap between parents and professionals, produced by misunderstanding, with a collaboration model. Today we struggle with the larger issues of supporting adaptation of individuals different from conventional social norms, individuals who with appropriate education, training and acceptance, can make valuable and often creative contributions to the larger society. This volume details some of the specific ways this is being carried out.

REFERENCES

Allport, G. (1966). ABC's of scapegoating. Anti-defamation League.

Campbell, M., Schopler, E., Mesibov, G.B., & Sanchez, L.E. (1995). Pervasive developmental disorders. In G.O. Gabbard (Ed.), *Treatments of psychiatric disorders: The DSM-IV* (2nd ed., Vol. 1). Washington DC: American Psychiatric Press.

Lovibond, S.H. (1954). The Object Sorting Test and conceptual thinking in schizophrenia. *Australian Journal of Psychiatry, 5*, 52–70.

Mesibov, G.B., Schopler, E., & Hearsey, K. (1994). Structured teaching. In E. Schopler & G.B. Mesibov (Eds.), *Behavioral issues in autism* (pp. 195–207). New York: Plenum Press.

Mesibov, G.B., Schopler, E., Schaffer, B., & Landrus, R. (1988). *Adolescent and Adult Psychoeducational Profile (AAPEP)*. Austin, TX: Pro-Ed.

Mesibov, G.B., Schopler, E., Thomas, J., Chapman, M., & Denzler, B. (in press). TEACCH transition assessment profile. Austin, TX: Pro-Ed.

Pollak, R. (1997). *The creation of Dr. B: A biography of Bruno Bettelheim*. New York: Simon & Schuster.

Reichler, R.J. & Schopler, E. (1971). Observations on the nature of human relatedness. *Journal of Autism and Childhood Schizophrenia, 1*, 283–296.

Rutter, M. & Schopler, E. (Eds.). (1978). *Autism: A reappraisal of concepts and treatment*. New York: Plenum.

Schopler, E. (1965). Early infantile autism and receptor processes. *Archives of General Psychiatry, 13*, 327–335.

Schopler, E. (1966). Visual versus tactual receptor preference in normal and schizophrenic children. *Journal of Abnormal Psychology, 71*, 108–114.

Schopler, E. (1971). Parents of psychotic children as scapegoats. *Journal of Contemporary Psychotherapy, 4*, 17–22.

Schopler, E. (1993). The anatomy of a negative role model. In G. G. Brannigan & M. R. Merrens (Eds.), *The undaunted psychologist: Adventures in research.* (pp. 173–186). Philadelphia: Temple University Press.

Schopler, E. (1995). *Parent survival manual: A guide to autism crisis resolution.* New York: Plenum Press.

Schopler, E., Brehm, S.S., Kinsbourne, M., & Reichler, R.J. (1971). Effect of treatment structure on development in autistic children. *Archives of General Psychiatry, 24*, 415–421.

Schopler, E., Lansing, M.D., & Marcus, L.M. (in press). *Psychoeducational Profile 3rd edition (PEP-3).* Austin, TX: Pro-Ed.

Schopler, E. & Loftin, J. (1969a). Thinking disorders in parents of young psychotic children. *Journal of Abnormal Psychology, 74*, 281–287.

Schopler, E. & Loftin, J. (1969b). Thought disorders in parents of psychotic children: A function of test anxiety. *Archives of General Psychiatry, 20*, 174–181.

Schopler, E. & Mesibov, G.B. (2000). Cross-cultural priorities in developing autism services. *International Journal of Mental Health, 29*, 3–21.

Schopler, E., Mesibov, G.B., & Hearsey, K. (1995). Structured teaching in the TEACCH system. In E. Schopler & G.B. Mesibov (Eds.), *Learning and cognition in autism* (pp. 243–268). New York: Plenum Press.

Schopler, E. & Reichler, R.J. (1971). Parents as cotherapists in the treatment of psychotic children. *Journal of Autism and Childhood Schizophrenia, 1*, 87–102.

Schopler, E. & Reichler, R.J. (1972). How well do parents understand their own psychotic child? *Journal of Autism and Childhood Schizophrenia, 2*, 387–400.

Schopler, E. & Reichler, R.J. (1979). *Individualized assessment and treatment for developmentally disabled children: Vol. 1. Psychoeducational Profile.* Baltimore: University Park Press.

Schopler, E., Reichler, R. J., Bashford, A., Lansing, M.D., & Marcus, L.M. (1990). *Psychoeducational Profile Revised (PEP-R).* Austin, TX: Pro-Ed.

Schopler, E., Reichler, R. J., DeVellis, R., & Daly, K. (1980). Toward objective classification of childhood autism: Childhood Autism Rating Scale (CARS). *Journal of Autism and Developmental Disorders, 10*, 91–103.

Schopler, E., Reichler, R.J., & Renner, B.R. (1988). *The Childhood Autism Rating Scale (CARS).* Los Angeles: Western Psychological Services.

Schopler, E., Rutter, M., & Chess, S. (1979). Editorial: Change of journal scope and title. *Journal of Autism and Developmental Disorders, 9*, 1–10.

Watson, L., Lord, C., Schaffer, B., & Schopler, E. (1989). *Teaching spontaneous communication to autistic and developmentally handicapped children.* Austin, TX: Pro-Ed.

CHAPTER 2

Core Values of the TEACCH Program

BACKGROUND

Several years ago at our University of North Carolina-Chapel Hill University Day observance, the keynote speaker, Dr. Robert Allen, described a Stanford University Business School study designed to identify shared elements of excellent and visionary companies. The authors of this study had assumed that the important variables would be factors such as exceptional leadership, strategic planning, mission statements, profit margins, or some combination of these. Instead, they found that what distinguished excellent companies was a shared core ideology: a set of values and sense of purpose beyond just making money. Moreover, those values were clearly articulated and well-understood among the workers of the companies. The core values were not the same from company to company, although they did have some important factors in common, but they all resulted in progressive growth and excellence.

In considering Dr. Allen's talk, I (Gary Mesibov) began to realize that TEACCH fits the pattern of the progressive organizations he was describing. That assessment was based on my personal experiences with this program, spanning almost three decades, plus the feedback that I get from many visitors and other outsiders from all over the world. These 'outsiders' frequently highlight the spirit and philosophy of TEACCH, which, in their opinions, both enrich and transcend the specific assessment instruments, conceptualizations of autism spectrum disorders (ASD), educational strategies, and therapeutic interventions we have developed.

In order to pursue my interest in having our core values be as clearly articulated and widely understood as possible, I recently sent out a questionnaire to ask staff in our program what they saw as our core values. The responses were immediate and enthusiastic. The following is my synthesis and prioritization of the five core values of the TEACCH program.

CORE VALUES

1. Understanding and appreciating people with autism spectrum disorders are our highest priorities. Although this is a relatively simple phrase, it has several components and profound implications. As I travel around the country and throughout the world, this is indeed the most important element others point to that consistently separates us from other programs. Similarly, in our North Carolina clinics, when therapists have become frustrated during collaboration with another agency, they invariably describe the problem as a lack of understanding, among the other agency's staff, of the client's autism.

One aspect of this core value is that we have a useful conceptualization of the communalities among people with autism that are different from other people. We refer to this as the Culture of Autism (see Chapter 3). Other programs often shrink from this value of analyzing and understanding autism, thinking that it somehow diminishes people with autism when we say they are different or not like the rest of us. In fact, I have heard TEACCH criticized for this reason. However, describing and highlighting differences is not derogatory. In TEACCH, we say that people with autism are different, and that is fine. Celebrating their differences, however, does not in any way limit our efforts to help them become as productive and capable as possible. In fact, *understanding autism is the foundation of our effectiveness.* One of our staff members offered several useful perspectives on this concept, saying "We work with autism and not against it," and that "We try to understand autism as another way to view life," and describing our mission as seeing life through the eyes of a person with autism.

Appreciating, accepting, respecting, and not judging autism are other important aspects of this core value. People from other states and countries who admire our work will frequently emphasize our respect for people with ASD as an important factor that separates us from other programs. One of our staff wrote, "It is important that we respect the perspectives of people with autism as valid." A psychology trainee wrote, "We accept limitations and we invoke the concept of grace, which offers our clients an endless supply of second chances." Again, respect for and acceptance of autism do not deter us from helping people with ASD to learn as much as they can and function as well as they can in our non-autistic, 'neurotypical' culture.

Finally, we really like people with ASD as people. One of our staff who is also a parent of a child with autism wrote, "TEACCH people like and appreciate people with autism. That really makes us unique and effective." Our enjoyment of people with ASD is seen in our appreciation of their idiosyncrasies and special interests, our delight in their humor, sweetness, and happiness, and our mutual pleasure in shared social events.

2. We are committed to excellence and have a strong work ethic. It was the commitment to excellence among our staff that originally attracted me to the TEACCH program when Eric Schopler offered me the opportunity to work for TEACCH, and that continues to motivate and excite me. When I look around the room at meetings with TEACCH staff, I see a group of wonderfully competent and motivated people who are never willing to settle for the status quo, but are always prodding themselves and encouraging, helping, and sometimes even prodding others and certainly myself to improve on what we are doing. Although it sometimes drives us crazy, I am very proud that we never rest too comfortably on our substantial accomplishments.

To me, excellence comes down to a simple concept, taught to me by my parents at a very young age and emphasized throughout their lives. I remember their encouraging me to higher levels of achievement when I would rather just slide along. The emphasis was always on my doing the very best I could, rather than worrying about the product, grade, or other symbol of achievement. If you do your very best with what you have, I was told, then everything else will fall into place. At TEACCH, as a program of people with many skills and talents in many areas, doing our very best with what we have results in exceptional productivity, creativity, and effectiveness.

Excellence involves persistence and hard work. Thomas Edison once wrote, "Opportunity is missed by most people because it is dressed in overalls and looks like work." We don't miss our opportunities. To be truly excellent, we not only have to do the best that we possibly can with what we have now, but we must also continue to search for new information and strategies to make all TEACCH services as effective as possible.

Excellence also involves challenging ourselves, debating with others, supporting our colleagues, rebutting our detractors, and defending what we do through our hard work and the products of our efforts. I do believe that any program receiving the national and international acclaim and attention that we do has to be doing something very well.

3. TEACCH professionals don't stand on ceremony or become overly impressed with their status, discipline, or position. There is a pragmatic, 'can do' attitude with a strong emphasis on getting accomplished what needs to be done. No job in our organization is too trivial to do well if it is worth doing. Interestingly, this was one of the more common of the core values that the Stanford study identified in progressive and successful companies.

I think this was one of the most important attributes of TEACCH that has made Eric Schopler emphasize the generalist model so forcefully. He remembered the days of interdisciplinary programs where each discipline worried only about their particular territory and the whole child and family sometimes got lost in the process.

One of Eric's most memorable stories was about a child with autism who was defecating in a vent in his house. After a thorough interdisciplinary evaluation, there were recommendations for correcting his articulation, facilitating his reading, diminishing his activity level, modifying his diet, increasing his peer contacts, flossing his teeth, and on, and on, and on. Although all of these were important and necessary, there wasn't a discipline that specialized in vent defecation, so there weren't any recommendations for the biggest problem of them all. In TEACCH, we attend to the vents if that's where the problem is (while also striving to make sure that whatever else needs doing is attended to as well).

4. A spirit of cooperation and collaboration characterizes all of our work. TEACCH was founded on the concept of parent-professional collaboration and this continues as a primary focus. Collaborations among our own staff and with families, clients, colleagues, students, community agencies, and everyone else concerned with people with ASD are also important goals throughout the program. Although there is the reality that one cannot always get along with everyone, this program values cooperation very highly and makes every effort to develop positive and cooperative relationships.

In response to my request for feedback, on of our secretaries wrote that "I feel this memo is exactly what the core value of TEACCH is, that you care to include me in this process. TEACCH has been successful in creating an environment where people work together." Others described our efforts to cooperate with even the most difficult agencies. One therapist wrote that "We work and function as a team without anyone feeling that they are an expert above the team;" another wrote that "In the clinic, the expectation is to ask for and give help freely." One of our job coaches wrote about the spirit of mutual support and assistance practiced at all levels of the program.

During these times when, according to George Carlin, people "laugh too little, drive too fast, get too angry . . . , when we have multiplied our possessions but reduced our values, when we talk too much, love too seldom, and hate too often," it is wonderful, even exhilarating for me to be part of a program where cooperation is so highly valued and so frequently practiced.

5. We look for the best in others and in ourselves. This is strongly reflected in our philosophy emphasizing the strengths and interests of people with ASD. This is also seen in the strategies we develop, and the ways that we interact with each other, and the many interested observers who visit on a regular basis. Various staff mentioned the importance of identifying and cultivating strengths as important TEACCH beliefs. One of our postdoctoral fellows described this core value as the belief that people with ASD can lead rich and satisfying lives. According to one of our therapists, there is always a feeling of optimism among the TEACCH staff and a striving to identify what is positive. When families feel despair about their child's disability, we value the need to instill hope about the future of the child and the family.

One of the most inspiring parts about this positive focus is that our program is able to maintain it without having to deny, minimize, or ignore the potential impact of this disability. We are able to accept and understand the reality of the condition and yet still see the strengths, courage, and skills in our clients, students and their families. For us, the glass is indeed half full, and we don't have to revert to false hopes to make our families feel positive about their possibilities. Our great president, John Kennedy, once described himself as an idealist without illusions, and I think we do a splendid job following in his distinguished tradition.

SUMMARY

We are, above all, a group of professionals and parents dedicated to understanding the disorder of autism, and in this quest we have found not only our life's passion, but a group of clients and families whom we admire, respect, enjoy, and genuinely like. In our work, we are committed to be the very best that we can and we are dedicated to doing whatever needs to be done for however long it takes in order to meet our lofty goals. In a world growing short of patience and respect, we try hard to support and cooperate with one another, as well as other agencies, and we maintain a positive perspective as we deal with a very severe developmental disability.

I have found identifying and articulating our values to be extraordinarily meaningful because it has reaffirmed why I work as hard as I do to be a worthy leader of our program and a public servant of the families from all over the world who count on us. I have enormous respect for the staff and trainees who share with me long days and the commitment to do the best we can to make the world a better place for people with ASD and their families. This exercise in core values has helped deepen my understanding of the bond that we share and the things that make us a team and a force throughout the world.

CHAPTER 3

The Culture of Autism

INTRODUCTION

Culture refers to shared patterns of human behavior. Cultural norms affect the ways people think, eat, dress, work, spend leisure time, understand natural phenomena, and communicate, in addition to other fundamental aspects of human interactions. Cultures vary widely in these respects, so that people in one cultural group might at times find those from another group to be difficult to understand or unusual. They might also evaluate their differences negatively, seeing them only as deficits.

Culture in the strict anthropological sense is learned: people think, feel, and behave in certain ways because of what others in their culture have taught them. Autism is of course not truly a culture; it is a developmental disability caused by neurological dysfunction. Autism too, however, affects the ways that individuals think, eat, dress, work, spend leisure time, understand their world, communicate, etc., and people with autism tend to be devalued because of their differences. So in a sense, autism can be thought of as a culture, in that it yields characteristic and predictable patterns of thinking and behavior in individuals with this condition. The role of the teacher or parent of an individual with autism is like that of a cross-cultural interpreter: someone who understands both cultures and is able to translate the expectations and rules of the non-autistic environment to the person with autism so that he or she can function more easily and successfully. To work effectively with individuals with autism, we must understand their culture and the strengths and deficits that are associated with it.

There are tremendous individual differences among people who share the diagnostic label of autism. The range of IQ's is a key source of this variability, in addition to age, temperament, interests, and the unique pattern of skills within each individual. From this point forward, we will use the term "autism spectrum disorders" (ASD) interchangeably with 'autism' to indicate that our concepts and methods are relevant for the entire range of developmental levels and behavioral profiles.

Because the organically-based problems that define ASD are not totally reversible, we do not take "being normal" as the goal of our educational and therapeutic efforts. Rather, the long-term goal of the TEACCH program is for the individual with ASD to fit as comfortably and effectively as possible into our culture as an adult. We achieve this goal by respecting the differences that autism creates, and by working within the person's culture to teach the skills needed to function in our culture. We work to expand the skills and understanding of the people with ASD, while we also adapt environments to their special needs and limitations. In effect what we attempt to do for them is what we ourselves might wish for when we travel in a foreign country: While we might try to learn some of the language and gather information about the customs of the country, such as the monetary system or how to use the telephone, we would also be very glad to see signs in English and have guides who could help us through the process of buying a train ticket or ordering a meal. In the same way, educational services for students with autism should help them to function more comfortably and effectively in society through two complementary goals: 1) increasing their knowledge and skills; and 2) making the environment more comprehensible.

To achieve these goals of helping people with ASD function more adaptively in our culture, it is necessary to design educational programs around the fundamental strengths and deficits of autism that affect daily learning and interactions. This approach to autism is related to, but different from, identifying deficits for diagnostic purposes. The diagnostic features of ASD, such as social deficits and communication problems, are useful in distinguishing ASD from other disabilities, but are relatively imprecise for the purpose of conceptualizing how an individual with ASD understands the world, acts upon his understanding, and learns.

We recognize that it is not possible to understand completely what any other individual experiences. We literally don't know what it is like to see through other people's eyes, and we can never know all of what another person thinks or feels. So our understanding of the culture of autism is necessarily incomplete and reflective of our own cultural perspective. Nevertheless, based on over 30 years of observation and close attention to the behavior and communication of individuals with ASD, we have established an understanding of various predictable aspects of the thinking, learning, and neurobehavioral features of ASD.

Following are the fundamental features of autism that comprise the 'culture' of this disorder. Most of these features are not unique to ASD; many of the characteristics observed in ASD are also seen in other developmental disabilities, such as mental retardation, learning disabilities, attention deficits, and language disorders. Some are seen in certain psychiatric conditions, such as obsessive-compulsive disorder, schizoid personality disorder, and anxiety disorders. Many are also seen in normally developing children, or even in ourselves. What distinguishes ASD are the number, severity, combination, and interactions of problems, which result in significant functional impairments. Autism is the composite of the deficits, not any one characteristic.

CHARACTERISTICS OF THE
CULTURE OF AUTISM

Differences in Thinking

The Concept of Meaning

A primary characteristic of the thinking of individuals with ASD, which separates them from the general population, is their difficulty imposing meaning on their experiences. They can act on their environment, they can learn skills, and many develop language, but they have limited independent capacity to understand what many of their activities mean. It is hard for them to draw relationships between ideas or events. Their world consists of a series of unrelated experiences and demands, while the underlying themes, concepts, reasons, connections, or principles are typically unclear to them. This severe impairment in generating meaning is related to several other cognitive difficulties, described below.

Focus on Details; Ability to Prioritize the Relevance of Details

Individuals with ASD are often very good at observing minute details, particularly visual details. They frequently notice when objects in their environment have been moved, and they may see tiny scraps of trash, threads to be pulled, flaking paint to be picked, drawers left slightly open, etc. Some also notice sensory details, such as the reflections of light, the sounds of fans or fluorescent lights, the feeling of fabrics on their fingertips. Individuals who function at a higher level of intelligence usually focus on more cognitive details, such as call letters of radio stations, area codes of telephone numbers, or license plate numbers of their acquaintances. What people with ASD are less capable of is assessing the relative importance of all the details they have noted. They might focus on the sight of the string they are dangling while crossing the street, and miss the approach of an oncoming bus; or they might enter a room and comment on the sounds of the fan, while ignoring the lighted birthday cake on the table.

The difficulty with meaning and emphasis on details lead to differences in the associations made by people with ASD vs. those made by their typically developing contemporaries. Most of us easily and automatically make associations in our minds that facilitate our understanding of situations and our ability to communicate with one another, but these skills are often limited among people with ASD. For example, a young man with ASD described the difficulty he had with following a conversation that went from red balloons to birthday parties to children having fun, because his only reaction to "red balloons" was his discomfort with the color red because it hurts his eyes. Another example was an adult who could not associate "Tiger Woods" with the golfer, because every time he heard those words he thought about tigers, woods, forests, and the wild. Even though he now understands what other people mean when they use that name, his thoughts still swing naturally to the two separate parts and focus on each of them in isolation from one another.

Most people in our culture assume that others make connections between ideas or events that are similar to theirs, which leads to many misunderstandings dealing with individuals with ASD. The teacher who assumes that her student runs out of the classroom in order to make her angry may be overlooking the squirrel that he saw, or the routine he has established whenever the door is open, or his enjoyment of the teacher's predictable response of running after him with a pink face. The parent who thinks that repetitive questions come from inattention or the desire for attention might miss the child's enjoyment of the predictability of the parent's consistent response, or the way a particular answer sounds, or how the parent's face looks when pronouncing the answer.

Distractibility

It is frequently difficult for individuals with ASD to pay attention to what their parents and teachers propose because they are focusing instead on sensations that to them are more interesting or important. In addition, their focus often switches rapidly from one sensation to another. Often the sources of the distraction are visual. For example, a teacher might put an extra pencil on the desk, and the child is so distracted by the broken point on the pencil that he does not attend to his work. Or the student sees something in the hall and is so fascinated that he stops working in order to watch more closely. Auditory stimuli can also be very distracting. A student may even be unable to concentrate because of a sound that the parent doesn't hear. Further, some individuals with ASD are apparently distracted by internal stimulation, such as a desire for the stick, string, cup, or other object that they remember from past experiences. Or they might be distracted by internal cognitive processes such as rhyming, counting, computing, or reciting facts they have memorized. Whatever the source of the distraction, people with ASD have great difficulty interpreting and prioritizing the importance of the external stimulation and internal thoughts that bombard them. Some individuals look, move, and explore constantly, as if all sensations are equally new and exciting, which for them they are. Others deal with this bombardment by appearing to shut out much of the stimulation around them, becoming preoccupied with a very limited array of objects.

Concrete vs. Abstract Thinking

Individuals with ASD, regardless of their cognitive level, have relatively greater difficulty with symbolic or abstract language concepts than with straightforward facts and descriptions. In the culture of ASD, words mean one thing; they do not have additional connotations or subtle associations. An example of this is a 15 year-old man with an average IQ, who was asked the meaning of the proverb "the early bird catches the worm." He replied, "If a bird wakes up early in the morning, he can catch a worm if he sees it and if he catches it, he eats it right up, and then he goes on and he looks for another worm." Similarly, when asked the meaning of "Don't cry over spilled milk," he answered, "If you spill milk you shouldn't cry over it but you should pick up a rag, you should mop it up and then clean the rag and then go have some more milk."

Another aspect of concrete thinking is that people with ASD generally interpret rules and expectations in a concrete, 'black and white' way. They have more difficulty with the 'shades of gray' that characterize social relationships in our culture (for example, 'little white lies;' teasing or flirting with peers vs. doing so with a supervisor; 'picking your battles' vs. constantly reminding those around you of what is 'right.'). A woman with ASD attributes her success as a computer programmer to her black and white interpretation of the world as matching the requirements in her field, where there are "no half-bits."

Combining or Integrating Ideas

It is easier for people with ASD to understand individual facts or concepts than to put concepts together or to integrate them with related information, particularly when the concepts appear to be somewhat contradictory. For example, a young man went on regular camping trips to a place called Camp Dogwood. Most of the camping trips were in the fall and early spring, never when the dogwoods were flowering. Each time this young man came to Camp Dogwood he expressed his wish to see the dogwoods flowering. Finally he got his wish when his group went to Camp Dogwood in April. Knowing how long he had waited, the woman who managed the camp placed a dogwood blossom on his plate, so he could find it when he came down for breakfast on his first morning. The young man picked up the dogwood flower and marched straight to the kitchen looking for the manager, not to thank her but to give her a long lecture about the inappropriateness of picking flowers and the importance of protecting nature (he was a member of an environmental club). When it was explained to him that she was a nice woman who had picked the flower as a gesture of affection, he insisted that if she were nice she would want to know that hurting the environment is wrong, so scolding her was doing her a favor. He could not understand how two inconsistent concepts (nice people save the environment and a nice person picked flowers) could both be accurate.

Organization and Sequencing

Related to the general difficulty integrating multiple pieces of information are problems with organization and sequencing. Organization requires the integration of several elements to achieve a predetermined end. For example, if one is planning a trip one needs to anticipate what will be needed in order to pack all of these items in a suitcase before leaving. Another example would be the need to collect all of the necessary work materials before successfully completing an assignment. Organizational skills are difficult for people with

ASD because they require the ability to focus on both the immediate situation and the desired outcome at the same time. This kind of dual focus is what people attending concretely to specific, individual details don't do very well.

Sequencing is similarly difficult for many people with ASD. It is common to see people with ASD begin a sequence, become confused, begin again or repeat certain steps, stop without completing the sequence, etc. Also, it is not unusual for people with ASD to perform a series of acts in illogical, counter-productive order, yet seem not to notice. For example, a person might get up in the morning, comb his hair, then take a shower and wash his hair. A person making lunch might take two slices of bread and then put meat on top, instead of bread then meat then bread, as we typically do in our culture. Sometimes people put their shoes on before their socks. In these ways they show us that while they have mastered the individual steps in a complex process, they do not understand the relationships among the steps, or the meaning of the steps with regard to the final outcome.

Generalization

People with ASD often learn skills or behaviors in one situation but have great difficulty using these skills in a different situation. For example, they might learn to brush their teeth with a green toothbrush, but then balk at brushing their teeth with a blue toothbrush. They might learn to wash plates but not realize that the same basic procedure is used to wash glasses. They might learn the literal wording of a rule but not understand its underlying purpose, and so have trouble applying it in different situations. For example, a high-functioning young man used to go into the building where he worked very early in the morning, to change his clothes. He was told that even though the building was open, there were still janitorial service workers throughout the building busily getting ready for the workday, and these people did not want to see him changing his clothes. He apparently understood this, but what he began to do was change his clothes out in the parking lot, in full view of everybody passing by. He honestly did not understand the concept behind the request, and thought that as long as he did not change his clothes in the building, he was obeying the rules.

Time

Many people with ASD seem to have difficulty with various aspects of time concepts. They may perform activities either too rapidly or very slowly, according to the standards of our culture. It appears that the concepts of "beginning" "middle" and "'end" are not always clear to people with ASD as they experience various situations, so that unpleasant activities seem to last "forever" or it is difficult to wait for things they want. Even capable adults with ASD who live independently are frequently late for appointments or have other troubles coordinating the different activities that comprise their daily schedules.

Differences in Learning

Several aspects of how people with ASD learn are also different in important ways from typical patterns in our culture. Considering these differences can be very helpful for people with ASD if we make appropriate adjustments in their educational programs.

Visual vs. Auditory Learning

People with ASD are visual learners (Quill, 1997). Temple Grandin (1996), a very successful woman with ASD, has written about her visual preferences with insight and clarity. She describes how her visual thinking facilitates precision in many tasks but makes conceptualization and abstraction more difficult. She also describes how she has learned to visualize more abstract ideas to help compensate for her difficulty. For example, picturing a child returning a wallet he has found helps Grandin to understand and remember the concept of honesty.

Prompt Dependence

Because individuals with ASD have so much trouble integrating information and understanding the world around them, it is easy for them to become overly dependent on others to provide prompts and cues to initiate tasks and complete established routines. This prompt dependence also contributes to problems of generalization. People with ASD can become so dependent on others in their environment to initiate and complete activities that they are unable to function appropriately or independently when placed in a different setting without adult facilitators available.

An example is seen in many young children with ASD who receive intensive one-to-one therapy to develop their language. Although this might increase the number of words they will say under highly controlled conditions with a one-to-one adult therapist, the child's prompt dependence is increased. For this reason the child rarely uses the newly acquired words in other situations with other people.

Differences in Neurobehavioral Patterns

Strong Impulses

People with ASD are often extraordinarily intense and persistent in seeking out the things they desire, whether these are favorite objects or experiences, or repetitions of an established behavioral pattern. These impulsive behaviors, which resemble in some ways the symptoms of obsessive-compulsive disorder, can be very difficult for teachers, parents, and the individuals themselves to control and channel.

Excessive Anxiety

Many people with ASD are prone to high levels of anxiety; they are frequently upset or on the verge of becoming upset. Some of this anxiety is probably attributable to biological factors. In addition, anxiety can result from frequent confrontations with an environment that is unpredictable and overwhelming. Because of their cognitive deficits, people with ASD often have difficulty understanding what is expected of them and what is happening around them; anxiety and agitation are understandable reactions to this constant uncertainty.

Sensory and Perceptual Differences

The field of ASD has known for many years that the sensory processing systems of people with ASD are unusual (Schopler, 1966). We see people with very unusual food preferences, people who spend their time watching their fingers flick, or rubbing textures against their cheeks, or listening to unusual sounds very close to their ears so that they can also feel the vibrations. We know people with ASD who don't respond to sounds the ways others do, causing others to think they are deaf when they have perfect hearing acuity. Some people with ASD seem to confuse the feelings of being pinched with being tickled, or appear not to feel pain at all. Others choose to rock back and forth for hours in repetitive patterns. In many different ways, people with ASD show us that their differences begin at the level of processing some or all the sensations that impinge on their body every waking minute.

MANIFESTATIONS OF THE
CULTURE OF AUTISM

The features of ASD described above interact to produce the familiar patterns of behavior characteristic of ASD. In analyzing the relationship of underlying features to patterns of observable behavior, it is helpful to use the metaphor of an iceberg. The tip of the iceberg represents the overt behaviors, while the submerged portion of the iceberg represents the underlying differences and impairments. We want to work on and change the behaviors we can see, but in order to do so we must understand the factors beneath the surface. Some of the most common surface behaviors and possible underlying causes are discussed below. Additional information about the manifestation of the Culture of Autism in individuals with ASD and average intelligence is available in Mesibov, Shea, and Adams (2001).

Attachment to Routines

A common outcome of the interaction of various aspects of the Culture of Autism is the need for sameness in the environment, which also presents itself as distress in the face of changes and disruptions in routines. This need for sameness probably derives from the combination of neuropsychological differences, heightened anxiety, problems with understanding the language-based expectations of others, problems with understanding the meaning and sequence of events, and unusual sensory experiences. The external world to a person with ASD is frequently confusing and stressful; as a result, routines and a predictable, stable physical environment are experienced as comfortable and gratifying. The person with ASD clings to them strongly, often expressing significant protest when they are disrupted.

Most individuals with ASD become easily attached to routines. Young children going to school might always want to follow an identical route to their classroom, touching the same door and greeting the same people. If the school secretary is out sick or they are asked to go directly to the auditorium rather than to their classroom, they can become confused and anxious. Another individual becomes agitated when snow requires an early dismissal from work or the Super Bowl cancels her favorite TV show. Strong and consistent repetitive patterns are deeply ingrained in individuals with ASD, who appreciate familiarity and repetition.

Tantrums and Aggression

Frequent temper tantrums are commonly seen among individuals with ASD, who might scream without apparent cause, destroy objects, or even attempt to injure themselves. In order to manage these behaviors, it is necessary to understand and attempt to modify the underlying causes, in addition to providing reasonable consequences. A major cause of temper tantrums in persons with ASD is limited ability to communicate. If individuals cannot express ideas like "I am still hungry" or "I have a blister on my foot," "I am ready to stop this activity," or "I am bored" they might be reduced to screaming and hitting. Similarly, if individuals do not understand what they are being asked to do or what is going on around them, they might scream or lash out. Tantrums are also often seen when routines are disrupted or the environment is changed, as described in the preceding section.

Occasionally people with ASD are aggressive toward others, even then they are not having a tantrum. Typically underlying this behavior are some of the same factors that underlie other socially inappropriate behavior. The person being aggressive might not understand that the object of his aggression feels pain. He might be attempting to initiate a social interaction without the language skills to do so, resulting in pinching, pushing, or slapping the face of the intended partner. Or the person might find the yelps, screams, or scolding generated by the aggressive behavior to be interesting on a sensory basis.

Limited Social Skills and Emotional Empathy

Social skills and judgment in our culture depend on the ability of the person to take multiple pieces of information from the environment, interpret and prioritize them, then organize an language-based and behavioral response based on an understanding of how it will be received by other people. Since skills in these component steps are all significantly impaired in persons with ASD, it is little wonder that their social interactions are frequently seen as abnormal according to the standards of our culture. For example, a youngster with ASD might meet a person in the hall who says, "Hi, Jim. What's new?" Jim might be struck by the pattern on the person's shirt, or be startled to see a person he was not expecting. He might not recognize that the words and inflection indicate a question, or might take the question too literally. So in response he might reach out to touch the shirt that was interesting to him, he might answer the question "I have new underwear" or he might offer a verbal reply like "what kind of car do you drive?" or some nonsense syllables that sound interesting to him. Such responses are understandable given Jim's 'cultural' background, but would be perceived as quite unusual in our culture.

People with ASD are at times said not to have emotional empathy for other people. There are several 'cultural' reasons for this. First, empathy involves feelings, which are much more abstract than facts or ideas. Second, empathy often involves understanding how another person experiences something, but to the extent that the sensory experiences of a person with ASD are different, it can be hard for him to relate to the sensory experiences of another person. For example, he might not understand or remember the sensations of stubbing his toe, bumping his head, cutting his finger, etc. Third, empathy involves holding two different ideas at the same time (that is, what I feel and what you feel) which may be difficult within the culture of ASD.

Limited Play Skills

One of the common sayings within the TEACCH program is that for individuals with ASD, "play is work and work is play." What we mean by this is that people with ASD generally have a much easier time learning how to work, which can be structured and organized for them, than they do learning how to play, which by definition is relaxed, creative, and less structured. Since relaxation and creativity are often difficult for people with ASD, it is understandable that learning to "play" is hard work for them, although it can be mastered.

Difficulty with Initiation

Some individuals with ASD appear to be "unmotivated" or overly dependent on a teacher or parent to engage them in any type of behavior beyond simply sitting or standing in place. They wait for prompts for everything: walking, picking up their cup or spoon, reaching for a toy, going through the movements for putting on a sweater, etc. Sometimes these behaviors are labeled by observers as "lazy," but in our view these surface behaviors or limited initiative can be explained by some of the underlying features of ASD. These individuals might have significant deficits in their ability to organize their behavior; they do very little because they literally do not know where to begin. They also might have very little cognitive understanding of either the expectations of the caregiver, or of the potential rewards that await them if they act. Further, because of sensory processing differences, the customary rewards for the behavior, such as the taste of the food, the sound of the toy, or a walk in the sunshine, might be meaningless or even unpleasant for the individual. Finally, the student might have an impaired sense of time, so that "excessive" sitting or standing as judged by a teacher or parent might seem like a brief pause to the youngster.

Noncompliant Behavior

Most of the behavior problems that people with ASD display are due to their cognitive difficulties in understanding what is expected of them or their overstimulation. It is rare, in our experience, for a person with ASD to be deliberately defiant or provocative. Unfortunately, some observers interpret their behavior as such, particularly when the individual with ASD looks right at them and then does the opposite of what was asked, or does what was just forbidden. In other individuals, we might rightly suppose that such behavior is performed to express anger or to assert independence. These are rarely the appropriate explanations for such behaviors by people with ASD, however. It is much more likely that the person does not understand the words used, or the facial expression and body language of the speaker, or the social expectations of the situation. Alternatively, the person might be driven by strong impulses to act regardless of rules or consequences, or he might be agitated and overwhelmed by sensory stimulation in the room, or the rules might be too abstract or too vague. Noncompliance is rarely a useful concept in ASD.

TEACCH EDUCATIONAL PRINCIPLES

Given the characteristic cognitive and behavioral patterns of ASD, the TEACCH program has developed educational strategies collectively called Structured Teaching, to help individuals with ASD function in the culture that surrounds them. (Specific strategies are explained in detail in Chapter 4, Structured Teaching). Structured Teaching is based on several principles, discussed below.

Careful, Ongoing Assessment

The notion of the Culture of Autism stresses characteristics and behaviors that people with ASD have in common, which are the foundation for the TEACCH program's Structured Teaching approach (see Chapter 4, Structured

Teaching). As in all cultures, however, individual members are also different from one another in important ways. In fact, people with ASD are probably even more different from each other than are members of other cultures. From the severely retarded, nonverbal child with problems of hygiene and aggression, to the high-functioning adult who can read, write, and spend time alone in the community, all individuals with ASD have gaps and skills, and all have potential for progress.

In the TEACCH program we supplement Structured Teaching with a highly individualized assessment process designed to identify each person's uniqueness. Observation of each person's approach to a variety of materials, directions, and activities, presented in different modalities with different amounts of structure, gives us important clues about learning patterns and understanding. We pay particular attention to the areas of communication, self-care, vocational skills, and recreation/leisure skills. Needs are prioritized and goals are established in each area.

The most fundamental component of this individualized approach is the assessment of how people with ASD understand the meaning of their experiences. Difficulty with understanding meaning is seen as the most central problem of ASD. We cannot ever assume that our students understand why we ask them to do some things, how the skills and behaviors we teach them are related, or even what, specifically, we are requesting. Even the most intelligent individuals with ASD are frequently confused or uncertain about expectations, social customs, and priorities. An effective teacher is one who can empathically, helpfully, and positively guide a person with ASD in our confusing and difficult-to-interpret culture.

Using Strengths and Interests

The TEACCH approach emphasizes appreciating and using the strengths and interests of people with ASD. For example, we can rely on an individual's attachment to completing tasks in a set sequence to teach the use of checklists for a variety of activities, such as personal care, household chores, vocational skills, and even leisure skills. Similarly, because people with ASD are very attentive to visual details, we can teach matching, sorting, and collating skills that can be used in real-life employment situations. Other examples are that if a student is strongly attached to the color red, the most important parts of his work can be marked in red; if his special interest is Star Wars, we can use Star Wars plots to teach writing skills and math skills. While we cannot change the autism, we can use it as a context to teach the skills required by our culture. Of course, all programs should work on both strengths and deficits to some extent, but the emphasis and priorities of the TEACCH program are clearly on strengths.

There are several reasons for this focus on strengths and interests. First, a competency-based model encourages more positive interactions with clients.

Deficit models tend to be more negative for everyone involved, repeatedly emphasizing what clients do not understand and cannot do. Second, building on strengths takes advantage of the unusual pattern of skills that is typically found in people with ASD. Although their deficits are difficult to erase, their assets (generally relative or even significant strengths in certain aspects of memory, visual perception, or unique talents such as drawing or perfect musical pitch) are easily cultivated. Moreover, their characteristic strengths in attention to details and precision are very much needed in our society and can be keys to successful adult employment. A third reason for developing strengths and interests is that people with ASD are much easier to teach if we are incorporating the things they are driven to observe, think about, or perform. Focusing away from strengths and interests often places teachers in adversarial positions with the compulsive interests and behaviors of their students. Why fight with these compulsions when it is far easier and more productive to incorporate them into activities to enhance their interest and enjoyment?

Family Collaboration

Educational planning should be sensitive to the environment where the student goes home at night, and will live as an adult. It is important to incorporate the wishes and lifestyles of the person's family into the educational program. For example, if the parents want or need the student to eat dinner with the family or occupy himself productively and safely during leisure time, we try hard to teach these skills. Consistency between home and school or day program is also important because it promotes generalization of skills learned to new environments, one of the most difficult, yet important, concepts for people with ASD to learn. While parent-professional collaboration has never been easy and is becoming more difficult during these times when so many are advocating litigation over cooperation, it is still one of the most important goals that can be achieved to help students with ASD lead more productive and independent lives.

CONCLUDING COMMENTS

Our goal as educators, parents, and others who work with persons with ASD is fundamentally to see the world through their eyes, and then to use this perspective to teach them to function in our culture as independently as possible. Although we cannot cure the underlying thinking and learning deficits of ASD, by understanding these deficits we can design educational programs that are effective in meeting the challenges of this unique developmental disability. "Structured Teaching," described in detail in the following chapter (Chapter 4) is the set of strategies developed within the TEACCH program for this purpose.

REFERENCES

Grandin, T. (1995). *Thinking in pictures: And other reports from my life with autism.* New York: Random House.

Mesibov, G.B., Shea, V., & Adams, L.W. (2001). *Understanding Asperger syndrome and high-functioning autism.* New York: Kluwer Academic/Plenum Press.

Schopler, E. (1966). Visual versus tactual receptor preference in normal and schizophrenic children. *Journal of Abnormal Psychology, 71,* 108–114.

Quill, K. (1997). Instructional considerations for young children with autism: The rationale for visually cued instructions. *Journal of Autism and Developmental Disorders, 21,* 697–714.

CHAPTER 4

Structured Teaching

FOUNDATIONS OF THE TEACCH
STRUCTURED TEACHING APPROACH

Introduction

The concept of structure has been fundamental to the TEACCH program's approach to working with individuals with ASD since its beginning. Eric Schopler and his colleagues, recognizing that the clinical approach of *unstructured* therapy based on psychoanalytic theory was unsuccessful, chose to pursue the opposite course. That is, the focus of their intervention efforts was developing highly structured settings for learning. The use of structure has continued to evolve in the four decades since the Schopler program was initially funded, and the TEACCH method of working with individuals with autism spectrum disorders (ASD) has come to be called Structured Teaching (Schopler, Mesibov, & Hearsey, 1995).

What is Structured Teaching?

Structured teaching is an array of teaching or treatment principles and strategies, based on understanding of and respect for the 'Culture of Autism' (see Chapter 3, The Culture of Autism), that can be applied on an individual basis to each person's particular situation. Specifically, Structured Teaching involves:

- An approach to serving people with ASD that recognizes both the characteristic difficulties of ASD and each individual's skill levels, talents, special interests, personality, feelings, quirks, and potential.
- Recognition of the needs of each individual with ASD for 1) visual and/or written information to supplement auditory input, and 2) some degree of external organizational support.

- Autism-specific supports that can be used to teach and support all aspects of life, including the development of communication, cognitive, self-help and daily living skills, socially acceptable behavior, social interaction skills, recreation, vocational skills (for adults), academic skills (for abstract learners) and participation in typical activities in the community.
- Autism-specific problem-solving strategies for preventing difficult behaviors whenever possible and dealing effectively with them when they do occur.

Structured Teaching essentially uses various elements of visual structure to translate the expectations and opportunities of the environment into concepts that people with ASD can understand, master, and enjoy. Parents, teachers, therapists, and others who use Structured Teaching methods function as cross-cultural interpreters, helping people with ASD understand the expectations and skills needed to function in our culture, and also helping non-autistic people understand and adapt to the needs of their students, offspring, clients, employees, etc. with ASD.

Structured Teaching thus has two complementary goals: 1) increasing the individual's skills and 2) making the environment more comprehensible and more suited to the individual's needs. In other words, some of the work facilitates changes in the individual, and some involves changes in the environment. To achieve the first goal, we introduce and have the individual practice new skills and behaviors. Of equal importance, however, is the work of developing situational modifications and supports so that the environment is in line with the individual's abilities and ways of understanding and learning.

Structured Teaching is appropriate for both children and adults, and is useful in a wide variety of settings, such as homes, schools, stores and businesses, camps and other recreational settings, job sites, residential programs, college campuses, etc. Structured Teaching is both a method for teaching new skills and a way of organizing any setting so that it is understandable and meaningful for an individual with ASD. The examples we will use in this chapter will reflect the range of ages, ability levels, and settings in which Structured Teaching is helpful. Additional information about the Structured Teaching methods with individuals with ASD and average intelligence is available in Mesibov, Shea, and Adams (2001).

LITERATURE RELATED TO STRUCTURED TEACHING

Both the research and clinical literature support the importance of structure and visual information to people with ASD.

Structure

Structure within the TEACCH program refers to active organization and direction of the physical environment and sequence of activities. Structure is essential to the functioning of individuals with autism spectrum disorders (ASD) because of their major difficulties with conceptual and organizational skills. The description of structure in a classroom used by Rutter and Bartak (1973) is still relevant and important today, and when generalized to a wide range of settings and ages is very much in line with the TEACCH philosophy. They wrote "By a structured situation we simply mean one in which there is a task orientation such that the adults determines what the child should be doing.... Whereas the normal child may well be able to profit by the opportunity to discover things for himself, the autistic child's handicaps impede him in this and he needs to be *taught* how to make use of opportunities.... 'Structure' carries no implications of rigidity or of rote learning. Nor does it carry any implication of 'discipline' or 'forcing'" (p. 257).

Research studies have confirmed the utility of structure as an intervention approach for people with ASD. As described in Chapter 1 (Origins and History of the TEACCH Program), Schopler, Brehm, Kinsbourne, and Reichler (1971) demonstrated that children with autism displayed more appropriate behavior in structured than in unstructured conditions. Similar benefits of a structured setting were found in the landmark study by Rutter and Bartak (1973) who were able to compare the skills and behavior of youngsters from three different educational units with different educational philosophies: 1) psychotherapeutic or "regressive" (p. 241); 2) permissive; 3) structured and organized, with more instructional time than the other settings. The students in the structured program were clearly found to demonstrate more on-task behavior and higher academic achievement.

Visual Information

The research and clinical literature also indicates that people with ASD learn and function more effectively using visual as compared to verbal information (Quill, 1997; Schuler, 1995; Tubbs, 1966). For example, a report on the "state of the science" (p. 179) in neuropsychological research (Dawson, 1996) concluded that skills in "visuospatial organization" are "spared" (p. 180), while impairments are found in many aspects of language and memory. Research has found that among people with ASD, a characteristic pattern of skills found on Wechsler IQ tests is having relative or absolute strength on visual-spatial construction (the Block Design and Object Assembly subtests) and particular weakness on verbal and social reasoning (the Comprehension subtest) although this pattern is not universal (Mesibov, Shea, and Adams, 2001). Grandin (1995), a woman with high functioning autism and a Ph.D., has described her cognitive style as "thinking in pictures." Hodgdon (1995, 1999) and Janzen (2003) have developed extensive educational materials based on the effectiveness of visual methods for supporting language development and appropriate behavior in people with ASD.

Numerous clinical research studies have also demonstrated the importance or utility of visual methods in helping people with ASD function more effectively. For example, Carr, Binkhoff, Kologinsky, and Eddy (1978), having taught four nonverbal children with autism to use sign language gestures for several common objects, found that "for three of the [four] children, correct signing was controlled solely by the visual cues associated with the presentation of a given object and was independent of the auditory cues related to the same object" (p. 489). Boucher and Lewis (1989) demonstrated that school-age children with autism made significantly fewer errors in response to written directions than in response to spoken directions. MacDuff, Krantz, and McClannahan (1993) reported that for four boys with autism (ages 9–14 years) living in a group home, "photographic activity schedules (albums depicting after-school activities) produced sustained engagement, and skills generalized to a new sequence of photographs and to new photographs" (p. 89). Similarly, Krantz, MacDuff, and McClannahan (1993) taught parents of three boys with autism (ages 6–8 years) to use photographic activity schedules, and reported that "the home-based intervention produced increases in children's engagement and social initiations and decreases in disruptive behavior" (p. 137). Pierce and Schreibman (1994) taught three boys with autism and significant mental retardation (ages 6–9 years) to follow picture sequences for various tasks of daily living, such as getting dressed or setting the table. They found that all children were eventually able to follow the pictures sequences to complete tasks independently, and they demonstrated that when they changed the order of the pictures, "the children followed the new picture sequence, suggesting that the pictures were controlling their behavior" (p. 471).

Visual methods have also been shown to decrease problematic behaviors (Mesibov, Browder, & Kirkland, 2002). For example, Peterson, Bondy, Vincent, and Finnegan (1995) presented data from clinical interventions with two school-age children with ASD for whom disruptive behavior and poor task performance were associated with verbal input from teachers. When gestures or pictures were substituted for the verbal input, disruptive behavior decreased and task performance improved for both individuals. Dooley, Wilczenski, and Torem (2001) described a "dramatic decrease in aggression and increase in cooperative behavior in the classroom" (p. 57) when a picture schedule was used to help a preschool-age boy make transitions between activities.

In summary, there is substantial clinical and research literature pointing to the importance of structure, the relative strength of visual processing skills compared to language processing skills in individuals with ASD, and the particular effectiveness of interventions targeted to visual strengths.

GOALS OF STRUCTURED TEACHING

Learning that Situations have Meaning and Predictability

In Structured Teaching, the environment and learning activities are designed to help people with ASD understand that the world is an organized, predictable place where they can succeed, rather than random events and disconnected objects that inevitably overwhelm or confuse them. Establishing a foundation of organization and predictability allows people with ASD to move

beyond their perception of fragmented details and begin to identify and understand meaningful connections in the world around them. For young children
and concrete learners, this predictability is the foundation for understanding
the routines of daily living, the language labels associated with meaningful objects, events, and people, and the power of communication to get needs met.
For older or more capable individuals, predictable situations help to make new
activities and expectations understandable and less stressful.

Skills for Adult Life

Skills and behaviors are targeted for their functional utility for the individual's future, rather than coming from lists of the typical developmental sequences. Beginning with even very young children, we teach the foundation
skills for as much adult independence and personal satisfaction as possible.
Important areas for skill development include self-care and daily living, communication, academics and vocational skills, leisure and recreational pursuits,
and community living. The specific skills worked on depend on the individual's age, developmental level, and cognitive potential, but at all ages and
degrees of skill we want Structured Teaching to build toward eventual adult
functioning.

Spontaneous Communication

An important goal is the ability to use communication spontaneously and
meaningfully. Some students with ASD must first be taught that communication
exists, i.e. that it is possible for a person to have needs met by influencing the
behavior of another person by some expressive act. The nature of this act can
be individualized for each person, with a range of options that include making a sound, ringing a bell, exchanging an object, exchanging a picture, saying
words, typing words, or using gestures or symbolic signs. Students having some
skills in communication can and should be taught refinements, such as additional vocabulary, more complex grammatical structures, expanded language
systems (such as written as well as spoken language), and pragmatic language
use in a variety of settings, including the advanced skill of conversation. (See
Chapter 6, Communication, for a more detailed discussion of communication
goals).

Independence

It is not sufficient to teach only compliance with a teacher or parent's requests, compliance with rules, or skills with materials or language, because
teaching a variety of behavior and skills that are unrelated, from the perspective
of the person with ASD, does not address the person's fundamental difficulties

with understanding, making connections, and generalizing. Unless a person with ASD genuinely understands what he is learning and how it connects to other parts of his life, that person won't experience the feeling of accomplishment that comes from mastery and that provides the incentive for continued exploration. For individuals to learn new skills or learn to function in new environments, teachers are very important. But ultimately we want people with ASD to be able to function without intensive supervision, because our culture does not provide resources for life-long teachers. Thus, the educational goal of teaching people to understand and meet expectations as independently as possible is both an important priority in terms of personal development, and a practical reflection of the general goal of helping the individual fit into our culture as an adult.

LIMITATIONS OF TRADITIONAL EDUCATIONAL METHODS

Because of the nature of ASD, traditional educational methods are usually not adequate for teaching individuals with ASD.

First, for typically-developing people, the simplest and most effective way to teach new skills and behaviors is through the use of language. For example, teachers in regular education classrooms talk all day long, explaining every facet of the skills to be mastered: how to ask for help, how to use scissors, how to write a sentence, how to solve an equation, how to write a term paper. Parents of typically developing children also rely heavily on verbal methods of teaching: how to act, what not to say, what will happen if they forget to do their chores, etc. Although verbal explanations and directions work well for most individuals, for those with ASD these methods are often ineffective, and occasionally counter-productive. This is true for people with ASD at all levels of cognitive skill. Even individuals with extensive expressive vocabularies often have limited ability to attend to or process a teacher's or parent's verbal explanations. For example, they might not know that they are being spoken to, they might be watching the pattern of the teacher's lips moving, they might be thinking about the sound of the fan in the room, etc. Even if they are paying attention, they may not understand language containing implied or dual meanings, idioms, complex structure, or abstract concepts. Individuals who have mental retardation in addition to ASD are even less likely to be able to learn effectively through verbal means. This is not to say that teachers and parents should not use language as one educational modality, only that reliance on this modality alone will probably be unproductive and frustrating for both the person with ASD and the teacher or parent.

Second, along with verbal instructions in our culture, we often demonstrate to our learners what we want them to do. Unfortunately, this technique is significantly less effective for individuals with ASD, because it depends on the person's ability to identify and copy the relevant aspects of the demonstration. For example, a teacher or parent might want John to imitate the way another student uses his knife and fork. But John might think that the concept being taught is having a striped shirt like the other student, or making the same noises he did. He might not be watching at the critical moment when the behavior is being demonstrated. He might see the other person's behavior, but have no idea how to organize his own behavior to look the same way. And of course he may have no idea what the teacher has said, or whom he is supposed to be watching. So while demonstrations have the advantage of being nonverbal, and are sometimes useful with our population, they are often not reliable or sufficient as an educational method.

Finally, in our culture we generally reward students' achievements with social responses, such as praise, smiles, pats on the back, and other acts that communicate "You have done a great job" or "I am proud of you." The effectiveness of these acts depends on the ability of the learner to decode the symbols of the teacher's pleasure, and on the meaningfulness to the student of the teacher's pride. But an individual with ASD may not understand the communicative intent of a smile, a sticker, a 'thumbs up' etc. or may not find a teacher's expressions of satisfaction to be relevant or meaningful. Overall, social reinforcement often has limited effectiveness with our students. We usually provide it, but we must use other methods in addition.

The difficulties that individuals with ASD have in learning from traditional educational techniques most certainly do *not* mean that they are incapable of learning, or that no effective educational techniques exist. The limitations of traditional techniques simply mean that different techniques must be adopted. In the following section we outline the elements of Structured Teaching for learners with ASD.

ELEMENTS OF STRUCTURED TEACHING

The elements of Structured Teaching are 1) Organization of the physical environment; 2) A predictable sequence of activities; 3) Visual schedules; 4) Routines with flexibility; 5) Work/activity systems; and 6) Visually structured activities.

Organization of the Physical Environment

Physical structure and organization of all settings should make them clear, interesting, and manageable for individuals with ASD—but the degree and type of physical organization differs among individuals.

School

For young children and concrete learners in self-contained special education classes, developing an appropriate physical layout of the classroom is an essential first step in assuring that it will be conducive to the needs, learning styles, and sensory differences of students with ASD. These students need visual organization telling them what activity occurs in each specific part of the classroom and also physical boundaries marking the areas. Physical organization generally involves the placement of furniture so that each student's ability to understand the environment and function effectively is maximized. Organization and placement of furniture can decrease stimulation, limit distractions, reduce anxiety, and promote independence and more consistent and effective work. Factors to be considered include sources of noise (such as the hallway, intercom, and other children), sources of visual distraction (such as windows, hallways, play area), efficient traffic patterns (direct path from one work area to another), proximity to a bathroom, and barriers that interfere with the movement of children who tend to run out of the room.

Visual cues can also be used to support physical structure. For example, important parts of the classroom can also be labeled with words, if these are meaningful to the students. Color-coding or labeling materials is another useful way of highlighting each individual's work area, which towels to use, where to sit at the lunch table, etc.

Higher-functioning students often can manage effectively in regular education classrooms, but there are some considerations related to the physical organization that are important for these students as well. Many need to have the areas where they work in the classroom be places where there is a minimum of activity or distractions. It is helpful for them to have an additional quiet area (or 'safe haven') to go to when the noise, visual stimulation, or their own level of anxiety become too difficult for them to cope with.

Ages of the students are another factor in considering physical organization in school settings. Younger students need areas for play, independent and individual work, snack, areas for developing self-help skills, and often a bathroom for toilet training. For older children, it is important to have places where they can pursue their leisure interests, develop vocational skills, and practice domestic and self-help skills, along with independent and individual work areas, places for group activities, and areas for whole class teaching.

Irrespective of students' levels of functioning, all educational materials should be clearly marked and appropriate for individual levels of understanding. Materials appropriate for specific activities should be available in the places where those activities occur, because easy access to materials when and where they are likely to be used is important for promoting independent skills.

Other Settings

Physical organization is equally important in other settings, such as homes and job sites. Young and very delayed youngsters with ASD often do not have an automatic or clear understanding of where they are supposed to be, and may wander from room to room. If they are not provided with clear physical boundaries, it is understandable that they might not learn our culture's expectations for being in the right place at the right time, behaving instead as though "we eat anywhere, we play anywhere, we get dressed anywhere, we sleep anywhere." Even older and more capable individuals benefit from explicit visual cues or written information about where to stand or sit, where to find supplies, how to get from one location to another, etc.

Predictable Sequence of Activities

A fundamental principle of Structured Teaching is that the sequence of activities is predictable for the individual with ASD. Predictability helps the person understand his environment and also reduces the anxiety that can be caused by uncertainty and surprise, which are particularly problematic for people with ASD. Predictability is especially important for students with ASD in sequential activities because sequential processes are difficult for them to grasp and remember. In school, predictability requires a schedule of learning activities for the day. A pre-planned sequence of steps can similarly be used for recreational activities, for therapy sessions (speech therapy, occupational therapy, even psychotherapy), for community errands, for household chores, etc. Although home life is typically not highly structured for most people, sometimes a home schedule is advisable, if individuals have difficulty occupying themselves during unstructured time or if the family is struggling with behavioral issues at home. In all settings, the sequence of activities is communicated to the individual with ASD through visual means.

Visual Schedules

There are multiple reasons for the use of visual means to communicate the sequence of upcoming activities or events. First, if the adult simply tells the individual what to do or what will happen next, the language might not be fully understood or might be forgotten, but visual communication is more likely to be comprehensible and can remain accessible.

Second, visual schedules can facilitate the transitions that often are so difficult for individuals with ASD and result in many behavioral difficulties. Following the familiar routine of looking at a schedule to understand what is coming next during a transition generally reduces the inappropriate behaviors that are caused by disrupted expectations and confusing or unwelcome interruptions in activities and changes in location.

Third, visual schedules help people with ASD to achieve the primary goal of becoming as independent as possible of adult cues and prompts. Because visual information is what they are most likely to understand, having individuals with ASD look to their visual schedule for this information to go from activity to activity maximizes the chances that they will not need additional prompting from adults. Teaching youngsters with ASD to follow visual or written schedules makes supervision more efficient for parents and teachers and also promotes feelings of security, competence, and independence in the youngsters.

A 'visual' schedule can take many forms, depending on the skills and understanding of the individual learner. Some youngsters develop reading skills and can use written checklists of activities for the day, a method not significantly different from those used by typically developing people to keep themselves organized. Many less capable individuals can learn to understand and follow schedules involving simple pictures or photographs. A simpler system involving a concrete object to indicate 'what comes next' can be used with the youngest and most concrete learners. (See Chapter 6, Communication, for a more detailed discussion of this topic).

Schedules can and generally should include times for free choice by the individual, because making choices strengthens communication skills, increases the person's willingness to cooperate with the schedule, and provides the person with control and pleasure. Schedules can actually make choices *more* meaningful to learners with ASD, because they can understand exactly what options are available.

Once individuals have begun to understand and follow a visual schedule, changes should be introduced into the content of the schedule. The schedule should not be the same every day, and pre-planned schedules should sometimes be deliberately changed in order to help the person learn that changes are tolerable. We do *not* want people with ASD to become attached to a routine; we want them to understand the schedule so that they can rely on it. Our goal is that people with ASD accept changes in the environment because they can rely on the visual schedule to communicate what is going to happen and in what sequence.

Structured Teaching classrooms simultaneously use two kinds of schedules: the general classroom schedule and the individual student schedules. A general classroom schedule outlines the activities for the entire class. It does not indicate specific work activities for individual students, but shows general work times (including the overall IEP areas that are being addressed, such as academic skills, self-help skills, domestic chores, or jobs around the school), snack, lunch, special classes like music or art, outdoor activities, etc. General classroom schedules are relatively consistent from week to week, except when there are field trips, special events, school assemblies, or other special classroom programs.

Individual schedules are designed for each person separately. For more skilled people with ASD, daily schedules are similar to 'to do' lists or appointment books that most people use. They typically show the entire day and have slots for each time period where the specific activity for that interval is written, along with a way to cross out or check off each activity when it is finished (for example, "science, PE, language arts, lunch, Spanish, math, homeroom). For individuals who have difficulty understanding written words, schedules can consist of drawings or photographs, objects, or whatever is at their level of understanding. For example, a picture of a desk or table might represent work time, while a picture of a swing might represent outdoor time, toilet paper might be used to indicate bathroom, a floppy disk might be the sign that it is time to use the computer, and a backpack might suggest the time to go home.

For individuals whose conceptual or organizational problems make a full day schedule hard to understand, their schedules could be presented to them one-half day at a time, or a few activities at a time, or even just one activity at a time. The important thing is that the type of schedule and the number of items presented are at the student's level of understanding and organization.

Routines and Flexibility

We encourage the use of routines for two main reasons. First, routines give individuals with ASD another strategy (in addition to visual schedules) for understanding and predicting the events around them, which generally decreases agitation and assists in skill development. Second, if parents or teachers do not provide routines, very often people with ASD develop their own, which are generally less adaptive or acceptable. For example, an individual might develop a routine of entering a classroom or work setting and touching all the coats on the coat rack, or might insist on smelling all the spoons set out on the lunch table, because that is what he did the first time he was there. However, if we teach a routine of entering the room and going directly to the puzzle table, or coming to the lunch table with a spoon already in hand and lunch already on the plate, the previous routines can often be disrupted and eventually forgotten, or even better, will never develop in the first place. Routines are especially helpful during transitions because these are the times that are most challenging for individuals with autism, when behavioral difficulties tend to occur.

The routines taught should also incorporate an element of flexibility because this reflects the reality of our culture. Our world is not invariable, which is what makes it so confusing to the person with ASD. The person's attachment to routines should be respected but gently challenged, for example through the use of slightly different materials for work, paths taken for walks, games played, food presented, times and destinations for community outings, etc. The essential structure of the routine should remain predictable, but details should vary, so that the individual is led to focus on the overall structure rather than on the details.

Structured Work/Activity Systems

Together, the schedule and the physical organization of the setting indicate the sequence of activities during the day and where to go for each activity. Once the individual gets to the specified area for the activity, it is the work/activity system that tells him what to do. Work/activity systems are critical for enabling people with ASD to understand the task or activity, stay focused, and complete the task independently.

Individual work/activity systems are organizational systems that provide the answers to four related questions: 1) *What* task or activity the person is supposed to engage in? 2) *How much* work (or how many tasks) is required during the specific work period, *or how long* will the activity last? 3) How will the person know that *progress* is being made, *and* that the activity is *finished?* 4) *What happens next* after the work or activity is completed?

Like schedules, work/activity systems are presented visually at a level that each individual can understand. A more capable person with ASD might have a written system with a written list of tasks labeled in words (such as "math, social studies, handwriting", or "sort, alphabetize, file"). The individual would know *what* to do based on the written words corresponding to the labels on each of the books, folders, baskets or other containers in the work area. *How much* work would be seen by the number of items written on the work/activity system or by a written indication of the time the activity session will end. The person would see that *progress* was being made as each of the written labels was carried out and crossed off. When all the labels were crossed off, that would be the sign that the work was *finished*. A written explanation of what would *happen next* would also be part of the work/activity system.

For an individual who cannot understand language easily, the four questions can be answered in other ways. A work/activity system for a more concrete learner might use pictures, symbols, colors, numbers, or objects. For example, a person at this level might have a work/activity system consisting of different colors secured on a Velcro strip going from top to bottom on his worktable. Each color would correspond to a color on a box containing a task. The person would know *what* task to do by matching the color from the work/activity system to the box with the same color (which would have a small piece of Velcro on top so that the work/activity system piece would remain in place). The person would know *how much* by the number of colored circles on the worktable. For example, if there were three circles, that would mean there were three tasks to complete during the work session. *Progress* would be understood by seeing the number of circles on the table decrease and the boxes moving off of the table into the finished area as tasks were completed, and the person would know that the session was *finished* when all of the circles had been removed from the work/activity system on the worktable. The activity that would *happen next* after the successful completion of the tasks would be indicated by a picture at the bottom of the work/activity system (for example, a picture of a computer activity, the snack area, a puzzle or magazine in the leisure area, etc.). More examples of work/activity systems and tasks (with photographs) are available in *Visually Structured Tasks: Independent Activities for Students with Autism and Visual Learners* and in *Tasks Galore,* both available from the Autism Society of North Carolina Bookstore (www.autismsociety-nc.org or 919 743-0204).

We typically teach following work/activity systems for completing tasks during 1:1 teaching sessions, using an individualized combination of demonstrations, hand-over-hand assistance, visual prompts, simple verbal cues, social encouragement, and desired activities at the end of the session. The tasks vary slightly, but the work/activity system remains constant until the person has learned to follow it independently. Then the work/activity system is used both in 1:1 teaching sessions to learn new tasks, and in the independent work area to practice previous tasks independently.

As described in Chapter 3 (The Culture of Autism), people with ASD have difficulty with finding meaning in many aspects of our culture, and in organizing and sequencing their behavior. Work/activity systems provide organized strategies for approaching a variety of tasks and situations in a way that makes them meaningful. They address the confusion people with ASD often have with 'beginning,' 'middle,' and 'end' by allowing them to see that they are making progress while involved in activities, and by making the concept of 'finished' concrete and meaningful, which helps people experience a feeling of satisfaction and closure when a specific activity is done. Work/activity systems also make tasks and events more predictable and therefore less anxiety provoking for people with ASD. They are also a marvelous tool for generalization because when the person has learned to follow a work/activity system, the system can be transferred to a wide variety of activities in a wide range of settings.

For example, we have seen work/activity systems used to show individuals

- How many subway or bus stops the person must sit through until it is time to stand up and exit the vehicle
- How to follow the steps involved in preparing a casserole before returning to a computer game
- The sequence of actions involved in scraping, rinsing, and putting dishes in a commercial dishwasher in a restaurant kitchen until it was time to take a break
- How to follow the routine of pulling down pants, using the toilet, using toilet paper, flushing, pulling up pants, and washing hands, then returning to the classroom
- How to follow the sequence of putting toothpaste on a toothbrush, brushing, spitting, rinsing, and turning off the bathroom light, then going outside to wait for the school bus
- How many helpings of food can be requested before the supply of request cards is gone, which means that the meal is finished, then going to watch TV
- How to complete a sheet of math problems, read two pages in a book, then write a paragraph about what was read, before having a choice of free time activities
- How many occupational therapy activities remain to be completed before it is time to go home

Visually Structured Activities

As discussed above, traditional education techniques for introducing new tasks and teaching new skills are often not very effective for individuals with ASD. We have found that because of the visual perceptual strengths of individuals with ASD, engaging them in learning activities can best be accomplished using tasks that are visually very clear and meaningful to them.

All activities for people with ASD should have a visual or physically concrete component. Language-only tasks are likely to be unsuccessful. If there is nothing for the person with ASD to see, hold, or touch, the activity will probably not be sufficiently meaningful to engage the person's attention for very long. Three aspects of visual information that help make tasks clear, meaningful, and comprehensible are 1) visual instructions; 2) visual organization; and 3) visual clarity.

Visual Instructions

Visual instructions help individuals with ASD to know what they are supposed to do. They are essential components of all tasks. These instructions can take various forms. Sometimes it is the materials themselves that show the person what to do, such as a sample of a completed block tower placed in front of him while he is working with a series of blocks (i.e. a *product sample*). Another common form of visual instruction is a *jig*, which is a silhouette, indicating exactly where items are to be placed. Because people with ASD like matching and puzzles, jigs can be a very useful component of visual instructions. For example, a jig of a fork, knife, spoon, and napkin can be used to show the person to select one of each utensil, and put it on a napkin; then the motion of rolling the napkin can be prompted and demonstrated. For more capable individuals, *written directions* are a very efficient method explaining exactly what is required and in what sequence.

Visual instructions are essential for several reasons. First, they help people with ASD understand exactly what they are supposed to do, using their strong visual-perceptual skills, instead of or in addition to their relatively weaker language skills. Second, learning to follow visual instructions supports the development of flexibility, which is otherwise relatively limited in ASD but which is so important for effective functioning in our culture. That is, if a person with ASD learns to complete a task in a specific way, it is often impossible to alter that routine or general approach to the materials. Through developing the person's ability to follow visual instructions, however, there is a mechanism for changing the person's approach to the materials when necessary. For example, sometimes the person puts clean plates on the table, but sometimes puts them in the cupboard. Sometimes paper is folded and put into an envelope, but sometimes it is shredded. Sometimes forks, knives, and spoons are sorted, but sometimes they are rolled together in a napkin. Sometimes putting on a coat means going home, but sometimes it means going for a walk. When an individual learns to follow visual instructions, changing those instructions can alter the responses and result in following different procedures with the same set of materials.

Visual Organization

Visual organization of materials also promotes learning for people with ASD. This usually involves evenly distributing and stabilizing the materials that are used in the tasks. Individuals with ASD are frequently distracted if their materials are not neatly organized and stable. They can easily be distracted or overwhelmed by sensory stimulation of disorganized materials (such as materials that roll around, fall on the floor, become covered up or mixed together). Since people with ASD usually have limited ability to organize their materials themselves, it is essential for teachers, parents, or other supervisors to organize the materials in an attractive, orderly, and minimally stimulating fashion. For example, in a sorting task involving a variety of materials, people with ASD are usually more successful and less anxious if the materials are neatly distributed in containers, rather than piled up on the table in front of them. Similarly, to teach a youngster to follow the morning hygiene routine, it is often useful to have visually distinct, separate containers for the various items needed for washing face and hands, brushing hair, and brushing teeth, instead of having all the equipment jumbled on the bathroom counter. For academic tasks, it is helpful to have each assignment in a separate folder, rather than having a wobbly stack of worksheets and books piled on (or crammed in) the student's desk. Structured Teaching settings typically have available a variety of organizational and stabilizing materials, such as file folders, baskets, trays, boxes, Velcro, two-sided tape, masking tape, etc.

Another example of visual organization is adding visual structure to a domestic task like cleaning windows. If the windows are large, people with ASD learning this task are often immobilized, unable to decide where or how to begin. Using masking tape to divide the window into four visually distinct square sections makes the space smaller and more manageable. This subtle but important way of providing visual assistance makes it possible for individuals with ASD to complete tasks that were previously too complex.

Visual Clarity

The visual clarity of the task helps students with ASD to identify its most important components and features. Tasks involving too many materials can be confusing or overwhelming, whereas tasks with a limited number of visually distinctive materials are easier to understand. For example, to teach sorting, a beginning task would use visually clear, distinctive colors or shapes (such as 'red vs. green' rather than 'red vs. orange,' or 'huge vs. tiny' rather than 'large vs. medium'). If a table is to be cleaned, scattering extra dirt or crumbs makes it easier to understand the purpose of this chore by magnifying the difference between clean and dirty. For individuals working on academic material, techniques to increase visual clarity include folding the page so that only the relevant or required items are visible, highlighting the sections they are to read, cutting and pasting items to increase the space between them, etc.

CONCLUDING COMMENTS

Structured Teaching is based on the assumption that programs matching the neurological needs and preferences of individuals with ASD will facilitate

their understanding and learning. Structured environments with strong visual
cues meet the needs of individuals with ASD more effectively than typical
language-based educational settings, because organized, visually clear environments and cues are more closely related to the ways individuals with ASD
process their environments. Structured Teaching helps people with ASD to
organize themselves and to function more appropriately, independently, and
successfully.

REFERENCES

Boucher, J. & Lewis, V. (1989). Memory impairments and communication in relatively able autistic children. *Journal of Child Psychiatry and Psychology, 30,* 99–122.

Carr, E.G., Binkhoff, J.A., Kologinsky, E., & Eddy, M. (1978). Acquisition of sign language by autistic children. I: Expressive labeling. *Journal of Applied Behavior Analysis, 11,* 489–501.

Dawson, G. (1996). Brief Report: Neuropsychology of autism: A report on the state of the science. *Journal of Autism and Developmental Disorders, 26,* 179–184.

Dooley, P., Wilszenski, F.L., & Torem, C. (2001). Using an activity schedule to smooth school transitions. *Journal of Positive Behavior Interventions, 3,* 57–61.

Grandin, T. (1995). *Thinking in pictures: And other reports from my life with autism.* New York: Random House.

Hodgdon, L.A. (1995). *Visual strategies for improving communication: Practical supports for school and home.* Troy, MI: QuirkRoberts.

Hodgdon, L.A. (1999). *Solving behavior problems in autism: Improving communication with visual strategies.* Troy, MI: QuirkRoberts.

Janzen, J. (2003). *Understanding the nature of autism: A guide to the autism spectrum disorders* (2nd ed.). San Antonio, TX: Therapy Skill Builders.

Krantz, P.J., MacDuff, G.S., & McClannahan, L.E. (1993). Programming participation in family activities for children with autism: Parents' use of photographic activity schedules. *Journal of Applied Behavior Analysis, 26,* 137–138.

MacDuff, G.S., Krantz, P.J., & McClannahan, L.E. (1993). Teaching children with autism to use photographic activity schedules: Maintenance and generalization of complex response chains. *Journal of Applied Behavior Analysis, 26,* 89–97.

Mesibov, G.B., Browder, D.M., & Kirkland, C. (2002). Using individualized schedules as a component of positive behavioral support for students with developmental disabilities. *Journal of Positive Behavior Interventions, 4,* 73–79.

Mesibov, G.B., Shea, V., & Adams, L.W. (2001). *Understanding Asperger syndrome and high-functioning autism.* New York: Kluwer Academic/Plenum Press.

Peterson, S.L., Bondy, A.S., Vincent, Y., & Finnegan, C.S. (1995). Effects of altering communicative input for students with autism and no speech: Two case studies. *AAC: Augmentative and Alternative Communication, 11,* 93–100.

Pierce, K.L. & Schreibman, L. (1994). Teaching daily living skills to children with autism in unsupervised setting through pictorial self-management. *Journal of Applied Behavior Analysis, 27,* 471–481.

Quill, K. (1997). Instructional considerations for young children with autism: The rationale for visually cued instructions. *Journal of Autism and Developmental Disorder, 21,* 697–714.

Rutter, M. & Bartak, L. (1973). Special educational treatment of autistic children: A comparative study—II: Follow-up findings and implications for services. *Journal of Child Psychiatry and Psychology, 14,* 241–270.

Schopler, E., Brehm, S.S., Kinsbourne, M., & Reichler, R.J. (1971). Effect of treatment structure on development in autistic children. *Archives of General Psychiatry, 24,* 415–421.

Schopler, E. Mesibov, G.B., & Hearsey, K. (1995). Structured Teaching in the TEACCH system. In E. Schopler & G.B. Mesibov (Eds.), *Learning and Cognition in Autism* (pp. 243–268). New York: Plenum Press.

Schuler, A.L. (1995). Thinking in autism: Differences in learning and development. In K.A. Quill (Ed.), *Teaching children with autism: Strategies to enhance communication and socialization* (pp. 11–32). New York: Delmar.

Tubbs, V. K. (1966). Types of linguistic disability in psychotic children. *Journal of Mental Deficiency Research, 10*, 230–240.

CHAPTER 5

The Theoretical Context of Structured Teaching

Structured Teaching, TEACCH's intervention approach for people with autism spectrum disorders (ASD), shares principles and techniques with other psychoeducational interventions for this population. For example, during TEACCH's earlier days in the 1970's when behaviorism was the predominant educational intervention approach for students with developmental handicaps, most of the TEACCH intervention efforts emphasized reward and punishment contingencies. This approach is similar to many programs based on Applied Behavior Analysis (ABA) today. Structured Teaching continues to share with ABA a highly structured learning environment that facilitates development in people with ASD. Unlike many ABA approaches, however, TEACCH does not create structure by relying on repeated trials that begin with a prompt and are followed by material reinforcements, because of concerns that doing so would likely lead to strong attachment to this routine (sometimes called "prompt dependence") and would compound already severe problems with generalization. Instead, structure is provided by the physical environment, organizational strategies, and the presentation of materials, which is also similar to the Montessori approach with typically-developing children. Materials are organized systematically in visual ways that are meaningful to individuals with ASD and are also tailored to individuals' strengths and interests.

Structured Teaching began incorporating perspectives from cognitive-social learning theory in the 1970's and early 1980's, motivated by the problems that students with ASD were having with understanding and generalizing what they had "learned" through reward and punishment methods.

Based on the work of Bandura and Walters (1963) and Mischel (1971), cognitive-social learning theory recognizes the utility of external rewards and punishments that characterize ABA approaches, but also emphasizes the role of internal determinants of behavior. According to cognitive-social learning theory, one's thoughts, expectations, and especially one's understanding of a situation have as much of an impact on behavior as rewards and punishments have. This additional perspective has become an important component in the Structured Teaching approach because the meaningfulness of situations for people with ASD is crucial for their ability to learn, understand, and most importantly, to transfer learning from one situation to another. The impact of cognitive-social learning theory has been that Structured Teaching emphasizes expectations and meaningfulness over contingencies, although rewards are still used and can be effective.

Making situations and activities meaningful for people with ASD is, of course, a challenge because they do not understand situations, materials, and events in the ways that neurotypical individuals do. Frith (1988) has written about problems with a lack of central coherence as the cause of many comprehension difficulties in ASD. According to this hypothesis, normally developing children and adults have a drive for meaning that enables them to pull pieces of information together to see and understand the larger whole. People with ASD do not seem to experience this same drive, so that their perceptions and cognitions are more fragmented and less related to one another. As a consequence, neurotypical individuals are better able to find and create their own meaning from individual events, while people with ASD do better with the specific fragments and details. As Claire Sainsbury, a young woman with autism, writes, "People with ASD have more difficulty seeing the forest through the trees, but we are able to see the trees with much greater clarity" (Sainsbury, 2000, p. 24). The chapter on Structured Teaching (see Chapter 4) describes how the TEACCH approach organizes environments and activities so that they are meaningful to individuals with ASD.

Perspectives from developmental psychology have also provided productive concepts for TEACCH and Structured Teaching. While cognitive-social learning theory led TEACCH in the direction of cognitive processes related to expectations, developmental psychology emphasized the importance of gearing experiences to the appropriate developmental levels for individuals. Development is frequently complex to assess in individuals with ASD because often they do not follow normal developmental progressions. It is essential, however, to understand each individual's developmental profile so that activities and expectations can be introduced at levels that will be most meaningful. If tasks are meaningful, they will be understood more easily, later practiced independently, and finally generalized. This perspective requires a degree of individualization of tasks and materials that is not seen in many other programs for people with ASD, which typically rely on one-to-one teaching of the same information and activities to all students. Use of a standard curriculum for all students is discouraged by TEACCH because each individual has his or her unique skills levels and learning pattern. Assessing developmental levels is an essential step in the process of developing educational plans.

Recognizing the importance of individual patterns of understanding meaning and of skill development highlights the need for more information about the brain and how it learns and organizes information in people with ASD. Accumulating evidence in the 1980's and 1990's has confirmed that people with

ASD have different ways of thinking, learning, understanding, and perceiving from those without handicaps. Understanding these differences has important implications for making instruction meaningful and understandable. In particular, recent advances in understanding visual thinking, executive functioning and the attentional differences in ASD have added to current principles of Structured Teaching.

Temple Grandin, one of the most celebrated adults with ASD because of her impressive accomplishments, has increased our understanding of the visual strengths of this group. In her book *Thinking in Pictures* (Grandin, 1995) she explains how she thinks visually, rather than using words and ideas in the same way as neurotypical individuals. Picturing visual images, rather than relying on words and ideas, makes her thinking very precise and enables her to excel in areas where visualization is beneficial. A disadvantage of this way of thinking is that because visual concepts are more concrete, the individual is less able to manipulate abstract ideas and concepts. This difficulty conceptualizing ideas and concepts, in turn, makes generalization difficult for people with ASD.

The results of a number of research studies converge to suggest that people with ASD process visual information better and are able to understand it more completely than auditory information (Hermelin & O'Connor, 1970;Quill, 1997; Shuler, 1995; Tubbs, 1966). Structured Teaching has utilized this information from personal reports of adults with ASD and from the professional literature to develop teaching strategies that rely heavily on the visual presentation and properties of information. By emphasizing visual information, Structured Teaching facilitates the thinking and learning of people with ASD.

Executive functioning deficits in ASD have been studied by several investigators (Ozonoff, 1995) who have documented difficulties and differences in brain functioning in the parts of the brain that control organizational skills, impulse control, changing sets, and related types of mental strategies. In line with these findings, the TEACCH program has developed and elaborated on several organizational strategies so that we can help children and adults with ASD to function better.

Problems with executive functioning and a related problem with sequencing information make it difficult for people with ASD to understand and follow the sequence of their daily activities. Not understanding what will be happening to them and in what sequence is a major source of anxiety and resulting behavioral problems. For this reason, visual daily schedules are an important component of the Structured Teaching approach. A visual schedule provides an individual with ASD, at his or her developmental level, with organized information about upcoming events and expectations, to compensate for the tendency toward disorganized, impulsive, or over-focused thinking and behaviors.

Having a schedule to organize the person's day is essential, but not sufficient. Executive Functioning deficits also interfere with individuals' ability to organize specific activities. Daily schedules get them to specific locations, but there is still a need to have a strategy about what to do and how to do it once arriving at that location. The second organizational system, the work/activity system, fills this need.

Research on executive functioning deficits in individuals with ASD has also enhanced our understanding of their difficulties with flexibility and changing sets (that is, making transitions from one activity to another). Rigidity and attachment to routines in ASD are widely reported and often acknowledged as a source of major difficulties. Strategies such as introducing changes in routines by making them very gradual and using familiar cues are essential for enabling people with ASD to function effectively in community-based programs with some degree of independence. Techniques for accomplishing this, consistent with neuropsychological principles described in the executive functioning literature, are described in the Structured Teaching chapter (Chapter 4).

Other important research examining neuropsychological deficits in ASD has been conducted by Dr. Eric Courchesne (e.g., Courchesne, 1989) who has written about the problems people with ASD have in switching their attentional focus. According to him, it is difficult to engage the attention of people with ASD and also to disengage this attention, once engaged. These differences from neurotypical learners in engagement have important implications; specifically, it is very important in all situations to engage people with ASD as soon as possible in meaningful, productive educational or vocational activities. When this does not happen, which unfortunately is frequently the case, individuals with ASD quickly become engaged in nonproductive, often disruptive behaviors like self-stimulatory activities, running or pacing around the room, disturbing others, etc. Teachers, supervisors, and other caregivers in unstructured situations often find themselves trying to disengage these individuals from such behaviors and re-engage them in more productive endeavors, a very difficult process to do with individuals with ASD given their attentional characteristics.

Understanding attentional difficulties has led TEACCH to pursue engagement as a priority, especially when individuals enter a setting and also during transitions between activities. These times are critical for avoiding the difficult combination of having to re-engage people with ASD after they have disengaged themselves from appropriate activities. Schedules and work/activity systems (see Chapter 4, Structured Teaching) have been developed to maximize engagement. Attributes of these systems that are especially engaging for people with ASD are the familiar routines they teach, the clarity and specificity of the systems and materials, the neat and orderly presentation of tasks, and the incorporation of the special interests of the individuals whenever possible. This emphasis on engagement, especially during transition times of the day, increases the likelihood that individuals with ASD will become involved in productive tasks and makes it less likely that they will become distracted, nonproductive, and disruptive.

A final concept that TEACCH's work with younger individuals shares with another approach is its child-centered focus, a strong priority that also characterizes Stanley Greenspan's "Floor Time" or DIR (Developmental, Individual-Difference, Relationship-Based Model; Greenspan and Wieder, 1998). Most other approaches to educating students with ASD are centered on theoretical concepts (e.g., making reinforcement the central component) or social-political goals (e.g., making normalization or inclusion the priority). For TEACCH and

Floor Time, however, the child is the focus, and all strategies and interventions are organized with the needs and interests of the child and family as their center. The child-centered approach differs from most other psychoeducational models, which typically involve developing a curriculum—usually based on normal development—and then encouraging, forcing, or otherwise trying to find a way to fit very different children into the same curriculum. In contrast, TEACCH and Floor Time build on each individual's unique interests, skill levels, and personal style.

In summary, Structured Teaching is an eclectic approach that incorporates several important psychological theories and traditions. The TEACCH approach reflects behavioral principles that are widely used in the field, expanded through cognitive-social learning theory and perspectives from developmental psychology. TEACCH also uses information from the neuropsychological literature that has increased our understanding of the thinking and learning process in all individuals and how these might be different for people with ASD. Individualization ("child-centeredness" for younger clients) rather than a standardized curriculum is also at the heart of the TEACCH approach. The resulting eclectic model called Structured Teaching has enabled individuals with ASD to function more effectively and independently in their homes and communities in North Carolina, nationally, and internationally (Schopler, 2000).

REFERENCES

Bandura, A. & Walters, R.H. (1963). *Social learning and personality development.* New York: Holt Rinehart and Winston.

Courchesne, E. (1989). Neuroanatomical systems involved in infantile autism: The implications of cerebellar abnormalities. In G. Dawson (Ed.). *Autism: Nature, diagnosis, and treatment* (pp. 119–143). New York: Guilford Press.

Frith, U. (1988). *Autism: Explaining the enigma.* Oxford, England: Blackwell.

Grandin, T. (1995). *Thinking in pictures: And other reports from my life with autism.* New York: Random House.

Hermelin, B. & O'Connor, N. (1970). *Psychological experiments with autistic children.* New York: Pergamon Press.

Greenspan, S.I. & Wieder, S. (1998). *The child with special needs.* Boston: Addison-Wesley.

Mischel, W. (1971). *Introduction to personality.* Oxford, England: Holt, Rinehart & Winston.

Ozonoff, S. (1995). Executive function impairments in autism. In E. Schopler & G.B. Mesibov (Eds.), *Learning and cognition in autism* (pp. 199–220). New York: Plenum Press.

Quill, K. (1997). Instructional considerations for young children with autism: The rationale for visually cued instruction. *Journal of Autism and Developmental Disorder, 21,* 697–714.

Sainsbury, C. (2000). *Martian in the playground.* London: The Book Factory.

Schopler, E. (Ed.). (2000). International priorities for developing autism services via the TEACCH model [Special Issue]. *International Journal of Mental Health, 29(1).*

Schuler, A.L. (1995). Thinking in autism: Differences in learning and development. In K.A. Quill (Ed.), *Teaching children with autism: Strategies to enhance communication and socialization* (pp. 11–32). New York: Delmar.

CHAPTER 6

Communication

INTRODUCTION

Disordered communication is one of the defining characteristics of autism (American Psychiatric Association, 2000). Since Kanner's (1943) descriptions of echolalia, literalness, and pronoun reversals in his young patients, and Asperger's descriptions in 1944 of unusual speech patterns, vocabulary, and lengthy monologues in his patients (Asperger, 1991), the communication difficulties of individuals with autism spectrum disorders (ASD) have been a major focus of concern and interest of researchers, teachers, and families.

This chapter will review the importance of communication in the lives of people with autism, summarize the research literature on the basic elements of communication development, communication disorders, and interventions in autism, then describe the TEACCH program's approach to teaching communication skills.

THE IMPORTANCE OF COMMUNICATION SKILLS

Limited social-communicative responsiveness and infrequent initiations of communication on the part of people with autism can discourage potential communicative partners from continuing to attempt to interact (Lord & Magill-Evans, 1995). It can be much easier for caregivers and teachers to do things for the person with autism than to attempt to elicit communication—and this is even more true for other children, who might quickly conclude that the child with autism can't or doesn't talk and therefore might as well be ignored. Clearly this can create an unfortunate cycle in which potential communication opportunities are reduced over time, leading the youngster with autism to be increasingly isolated and non-communicative.

The most fundamental reason to teach communication to students with autism is the same reason that communication is so important for all of us: so that we can get needs met as fully and precisely as possible. It is very difficult to know what other people want or what they are thinking, in the absence of communication. Is he hungry? Does he want peanut butter or cheese? Is there a particular toy he wants us to reach for him? Is he cold? Does he want to go outside? Do his shoes hurt? Does he want the computer or television adjusted?

In addition to these kinds of specific requests, some of which could eventually be identified through a trial and error procedure on the part of caregivers, another function of communication is to express a person's unique humanity. What is he seeing that strikes him as interesting or funny? Is he experiencing a feeling that another person could understand? Does he have thoughts, suggestions, or creative ideas that other people could share, benefit from, enjoy?

Further, those of us who do not have ASD understand clearly the benefits and pleasures of social contacts, and we want to teach social-communication skills to people with ASD so that they can experience these as much as possible. We know how much pleasure can come from playing a game together, sharing a laugh at a funny movie, or splashing each other in a swimming pool. When we can engage individuals with ASD in these shared social-communicative experiences, we enrich their lives beyond simple requests for food, drink, toys, etc.

Another benefit of communication is that individuals experience less confusion and helplessness when they can understand information from others. Through communication we can decrease the person's anxiety and discomfort. For example, we can explain what is going on (such as a thunder storm or fire drill), or what will happen next (such as a meal, going to school, home, grocery story, etc.). While these kinds of explanations are important for all youngsters, people with ASD are often particularly confused about the sequence or timing of events around them. (This is the reason they so often cling to known routines and become distressed at unexpected change.) We can help them be more comfortable if we can communicate about the sequence of events. By using communication to make the world seem more orderly and manageable, we support the individual with ASD to engage in and even look for activities and relationships (see also Chapter 4, Structured Teaching).

Similarly, uncomfortable feelings of frustration can be reduced when individuals can express their wishes in ways that others can understand. If he wants juice instead of water, playdoh instead of a puzzle, a new crayon instead of the old one with the torn label, etc., he will be much happier if his family and teachers can understand and accommodate his wishes.

Finally, by teaching individuals with autism effective means to express themselves and to understand their caregivers and teachers as much as possible, we can decrease behavior problems. Very often, behaviors such as crying, screaming, grabbing materials, repetitive questioning, or aggression are indications that people with autism are confused or frustrated by what is happening around them. By giving individuals with autism ways to understand what is happening and to change or influence it, we give them alternatives to tantrums, unusual repetitive behaviors, and other problematic ways of expressing their distress (Carr & Carlson, 1993; Carr & Durand, 1985; Durand & Carr, 1992; Frea, Arnold, & Vittimberga, 2001; Goldstein, 2002; Hurtig, Ensrud, & Tomblin, 1982; Koegel, 2000; Mirenda, 1997).

DEFINITIONS

Language is a formal system of symbols that two or more people understand and use to share information with each other. Examples of language are spoken English, written French, American Sign Language, and ancient Egyptian hieroglyphics. If you know the particular symbols, you can understand the information expressed by them, and you can use the language symbols to express yourself. *Receptive language* refers to language that is understood and *expressive* language refers to language that is produced. *Meaningful expressive language rests on a foundation of receptive understanding.*

Language is one form of *communication*, which is a broader category that includes other behaviors, such as simple gestures, facial expressions, crying and other sounds, and any other signals that intentionally send information from one person to another. Bates (1979, as cited in Wetherby, Schuler, & Prizant, 1997) defined communication as "signaling behavior in which the sender is aware *a priori* of the effect that a signal will have on his listener, and he persists in that behavior until the effect is obtained or failure is clearly indicated (p. 36)." According to this definition an act is communicative if the sender intends it to be, not just if the observer/listener interprets it as having meaning. However, others in the field (Wetherby et al., 1997) suggest that any behavior can function as communication, even if it is unintentional on the part of the sender. Using this definition, a baby's cry "communicates" hunger or distress to a parent, even if the baby does not yet understand this or anticipate the parent's reaction.

There are a number of aspects of language that can be analyzed separately. *Semantics* refers to the *meanings* of the symbols that make up the language. Thus, in English and other spoken or written language, semantics refers to the meanings of words. *Speech* is the production of the *sounds* of a language; other terms that have similar meanings are *articulation* and *phonology*. Another element of the sound of language is *prosody*, which refers to the *rhythm, intonation, and stress patterns* of speech (Baltaxe & Simmons, 1992). *Syntax* is the technical term that means the rules or *grammar* of a language. For example, in English the subject generally comes before the verb, adjectives come before the noun they modify, etc. Closely related to syntax is *morphology*, which refers to the small markers on words that convey meaning, such as '-s' for plurals, '-ed' for past tense, etc. *Pragmatics* means the functional *use* of language in context. Seibert and Oller (1981) described the relationships among these various factors: "If the training of syntactic skills is directed toward teaching a child how to say things, and if the training of semantic skills is directed to teaching the child to say things meaningfully, then the training of linguistic pragmatic skills is directed to teaching the child to achieve things by saying things meaningfully in appropriate situations" (p. 78).

RESEARCH LITERATURE ON COMMUNICATION AND LANGAUGE PATTERNS IN AUTISM

Over the past quarter century, researchers have studied these various aspects of the communication and language skills of people diagnosed with autism. The following points are now generally accepted in the literature:

Who Develops Expressive Language?

The proportion of individuals with autism who eventually develop some useful expressive language used to be cited as 50% (Konstantareas, 1996; Wetherby et al., 1997), but recent research, published since the widespread availability of special education and speech/language therapy services, suggests that the percentage might markedly higher. For example, Eaves and Ho (1996) found that over 80% of their sample (average age of 11 $\frac{1}{2}$ years) used at least 6 words to communicate at home. Koegel (1995) reported that of the 50% of children with autism who are nonverbal, 70% can learn "at least some expressive language" with appropriate "naturalistic" intervention (p. 18). Rogers (1996), in reviewing a variety of early intervention programs, found that 73% of the youngsters "had useful speech by the end of the intervention period (generally age 5)" (p. 243). More recently, Koegel (2000) has re-stated that "as many as 85–90% of children diagnosed as having autism, who begin intervention before the age of 5, can learn to use verbal communication as a primary mode of communication" (p. 384). However, as Lord and Paul (1997) pointed out, reports of expressive language usage do not necessarily reflect how often individuals speak, under what circumstances, at what length, or for what purposes. Some individuals have only a small repertoire of single-word expressions, some go for days or weeks without speaking, some repeat long sequences of television dialogue but rarely use language for typical purposes such as making requests or engaging in social interactions, etc.

Several recent studies have attempted to identify early developmental factors associated with eventual development of speech. Stone and Yoder (2001) reported that motor imitation skills at age 2 years and the number of hours of speech/language therapy received between ages 2–3 years were significantly associated with speech development by age 4 years. The authors discussed the importance of the predictive power of early imitation skills, indicating that "because of its social and representational components, as well as the relative ease with which it can be assessed, motor imitation ability may be a particularly useful early indicator of future language development in children with autism spectrum disorders" (p. 354). In this study, object play and initiation of joint attention at age 2 years were not significantly associated with later speech development, when speech skills at age 2 years were statistically controlled. These findings were somewhat different from the results reported by Sigman and Ruskin (1999) who found that responding to joint attention opportunities between the ages of 2–6 years was significantly associated with speech development at ages 10–13 years, and that early functional (nonsymbolic) play was also associated with later speech. Stone and Yoder (2001) speculated that the different findings might have been due to different measures of joint attention and different ages of subjects (with 2-year-olds having more variable, less predictable developmental trajectories).

The lack of development of speech by age 5 years is generally considered to be predictive of a limited prognosis for eventual independence (Lord & Bailey, 2002), although some children develop some speech after this age (e.g., Ballaban-Gil et al., 1996).

Do Some Children Develop Expressive Language then Lose It?

A substantial minority of children with autism (approximately 20–37%, according to various sources) develop some expressive language then lose it (APA, 2000; Davidovitch, Glick, Holtzman, Tirosh, & Safir, 2000; Goldberg et al., 2003; Kurita, 1985; Lord & Paul, 1997; Lotter, 1966; Mantovani, 2000; Shinnar et al., 2001). Kurita (1985) studied 97 of these children and found the following profile: most (94%) were using only a few spontaneous single words before the loss of speech. They had begun using words earlier than other children with autism who did not experience speech loss, although in other aspects of development most (78%) had showed some developmental abnormalities prior to speech loss. The median age at which they stopped speaking was 18 months; for 73% of the children this was within 6 months of when they had begun speaking, including approximately one-third of the sample who lost speech within one month of developing it. Kurita, Kita, and Miyake (1992) reported similar findings in a group of 51 youngsters with autism with an episode of speech loss. Goldberg et al. (2003) also found that typical age of language loss was 18–21 months, and that it was almost always accompanied or preceded by loss of other skills as well. While the reasons for the loss of language skills are not clear, Tager-Flusberg (1997) has postulated that the phenomenon occurs when children are at the very early language development stage of slowly learning to associate specific words with very significant objects or activities (such as bottle, outside, Daddy) but have not yet shifted into the stage of rapidly understanding and generalizing the meanings of words in larger categories. Thus, what appears to be a dramatic loss of skills may be better conceptualized as the failure to make progress to the next level of language development, along with the fading out of the memorized words.

What Interferes with Language Development?

Many of the individuals who do not develop expressive language seem not to have a well-developed understanding of the power of communication, and so they lack *communicative intent* (Prizant & Wetherby, 1987). That is, although they may have the oral-motor skills to produce sounds or even imitate words, some people with autism seem not to understand that they can influence other people by communicating what it is they want (Curcio, 1978; McHale, Simeon-sson, Marcus, & Olley, 1980; Prizant & Duchan, 1981, Stone & Caro-Martinez, 1990). These individuals find it easier to get what they want by themselves than to use communication to ask another person to get it for them. Without interventions that teach them the power and utility of meaningful communication, these individuals are at high risk of remaining functionally mute and socially very isolated.

Other individuals with autism appear to have specific *difficulty with initiating* actions. These individuals may respond to directions and initiations by others, but when left alone simply sit passively (Wing & Gould, 1979). This general difficulty with initiation can clearly be associated with limited initiation of communicative exchanges (Koegel, Koegel, Shoshan, & McNerney, 1999; Stone & Caro-Martinez, 1990).

Another aspect of autism that may interfere with verbal language development is *difficulty with sensory integration*, including processing sounds and verbal language (Anzalone & Williamson, 2000; Dawson & Watling, 2000; Kientz & Dunn, 1997; Lord & Risi, 2000). Many people with autism appear to be overly sensitive to sensory sensations, including sounds; for example, they cover their ears or become distressed by sounds such as vacuum cleaners, sirens, and crowded, noisy places. Others are so under-responsive to sounds that they were at some point suspected of being deaf. Some individuals even show both patterns. In addition, it has been theorized that children with autism process language in a gestalt or holistic fashion, rather than being able to segment and analyze individual words and portions of words (Wetherby et al., 1997). Overall, for people with autism, the auditory channel is less efficient and comfortable than the visual channel, so that hearing and processing language are relatively difficult tasks.

Research indicates that those youngsters with autism who do develop useful speech generally acquire this skill more slowly, and therefore later, than typical children. One reason for this is that the proportion of people with autism and co-occurring *mental retardation* has historically been approximately 75% (Mesibov, Adams, & Klinger, 1997), although the current figure may be somewhat lower (Bryson & Smith, 1998). Mental retardation means that the children's cognitive and adaptive skills are delayed for their chronological ages. These youngsters learn more slowly than typically developing children and need more instruction and repetition in order to master skills in all areas. Typically-developing babies listen to language for many months before beginning to understand the words; expressive language begins even later. In the same way, children with autism need to have communicative mechanisms associated with meaningful objects or activities for a substantial period of time before they begin to make the associations. The amount of time an individual child needs to learn each association cannot be predicted, but having mental retardation in addition to autism suggests that learning all cognitive skills, including communication, will be significantly slower than average. Delays in receptive and expressive language development may thus be one aspect of overall developmental delay.

The exception to the co-occurrence of autism and mental retardation is the autism spectrum disorder known as Asperger Syndrome or Asperger's Disorder (APA, 2000) also sometimes called High Functioning Autism (Mesibov, Shea, & Adams, 2001; Schopler, Mesibov & Kunce, 1998). This type of autism is not associated with mental retardation, and language milestones are met approximately at the normal time. However, even individuals with Asperger Syndrome/High Functioning Autism have disorders of other aspects of language development, including unusual prosody, limited understanding of more abstract aspects of language such as humor, sarcasm, and figures of speech, and difficulty carrying on a reciprocal conversation with another person (Klin and Volkmar, 1997; Landa 2000). People with Asperger Syndrome/High Functioning Autism generally do learn the mechanics of reading and writing at grade level, but some academic tasks, such as reading comprehension that involves abstract concepts or interpersonal relations, remain relatively less advanced (Minshew, Goldstein, & Siegel, 1995; Minshew, Goldstein, Taylor, & Siegel, 1994).

Are All Language Skills Equally Affected by Autism?

Although the focus of many clinical and research efforts is on the development of *expressive* language, it is important not to overlook the frequent difficulties with *comprehension* of language that are frequently, if not inevitably, present in autism spectrum disorders (Lord, 1985; Lord & Paul, 1997). As Lord (1985) pointed out, "Normally developing children can work back and forth from sentence to situation using what they know about the specific context as well as the general likelihood of events to determine which... [meaning] is intended." (p. 258). Individuals with autism, on the other hand, have difficulty using meaning to guide their comprehension of language. Thus, for example, Tager-Flusberg (1981b) found that a group of youngsters with autism did not use their knowledge of what is likely and probable to help them understand sentences such as 'the baby wears the hat' vs. 'the hat wears the baby.' Lord (1985) described children with autism as being "doubly handicapped" (p. 258) because in addition to having delayed development in language structures, they also have much less understanding of the world around them to serve as a basis for understanding language about that world. Even older individuals with relatively well-developed vocabularies may still have significant difficulty understanding language involving metaphors, double meanings, implied meaning, sarcasm, and word play (Landa, 2000).

In terms of expressive language, researchers have found that although most children with autism develop more slowly than average, the acquisition of some aspects of language generally follows the typical developmental path, while other aspects of language are markedly disordered (Konstantareas & Beitchman, 1996; Swisher & Demetras, 1985; Tager-Flusberg, 1994, 1997; 2001; Wetherby & Prutting, 1984).

Specifically, among those who do develop some expressive language, *phonological* skills (discriminating and producing speech sounds) generally emerge in the same sequence as those of typical children. *Prosody*, on the other hand, is generally unusual in some way (Baltaxe & Simmons, 1985; Tager-Flusberg, 1981a, 1997). Research on the atypical prosodic characteristics of people with ASD is summarized by Frea (1995) as including "flat, expressionless speech; rapid, staccato delivery; singsong intonation; errors in stress assignment; excessive high pitch without pitch changes; hoarseness, harshness, and hypernasality; vocal volume too high or low a level or varying intensity inappropriately; and incorrect primary sentence stress" (p. 56). Verbal children with ASD usually use *syntax* (grammar) that is comparable to that of younger typically-developing children and children with mental retardation, except for somewhat less complex spontaneous speech (Pierce & Bartolucci, 1977; Tager-Flusberg et al., 1990).

The *semantic* (vocabulary and meaning) skills of people with autism are often both delayed and disordered. The classic observation (Kanner, 1943) that children with autism confuse "I" and "you" is one of several indications of the common difficulty with words that change meaning depending on who is speaking; another example is "here" and "there" (Bartolucci, Pierce, & Streiner, 1980). Children with autism have also been found both to use unusual words and phrases, and to have difficulty understanding the meaning of what is said to them (Lord & Paul, 1997; Volden & Lord, 1991).

Another experimental finding indicating weakness in semantic skills relative to other skills came from the work of Hermelin and O'Connor (1970), who found that on verbal memory tasks children with autism were much less likely than typical or mentally retarded children to use semantic categories to help them remember a series of words (such as "blue, three, red, five, white, six"), apparently relying instead on rote memory. Children with autism have also been found to understand and use words related to social-emotional topics and to mental processes (such as "think," "pretend") less well than other children (Tager-Flusberg, 2001).

The most striking aspect of the expressive language disorder of people with ASD is in the area of *pragmatics* (Baron-Cohen, 1988; Lord & Paul, 1997; Tager-Flusberg, 1981a). Bruner (1981, cited in Wetherby et al., 1997) described three basic pragmatic functions of communication: 1) behavioral regulation of others (for example, requesting something to drink or protesting being touched); 2) social interaction (such as vocalizing to get attention); and 3) joint attention (such as pointing to something or commenting about it in order to share enjoyment of it with another person). Wetherby (1986) suggested that Bruner's list represents the sequence in which these pragmatic skills emerge in children with autism, with some individuals rarely, if ever, using communication for joint attention purposes. Even those individuals who have functional verbal language generally do not use it for the same purposes and with the same flexibility and social sensitivity as people without autism (Capps, Kehres, & Sigman, 1998; Eales, 1993; Fine, Bartolucci, Szatmari, & Ginsberg, 1994; Stone & Caro-Martinez, 1990; Tager-Flusberg, 2001; Twachtman, 1995).

Wetherby and Prutting (1984) identified other differences between the communication of groups of children with autism and typically developing children who were at the same stage of expressive communication development (that is, prelinguistic through three words). In this study, the mean age of the autism group was 9 years, 6 months, while the mean age of the typical group was 1 year, 7 months. During an hour-long observation session, the two groups did not differ significantly in the *number* of communicative acts emitted in an hour; in fact, as a group the youngsters with autism produced slightly *more* communicative acts. However, the two groups used their language for markedly different *purposes*. The children with autism mostly requested objects, requested actions, and protested. There was no acknowledgment of another person, showing off, commenting, or labeling of objects for social purposes. Other social-communicative functions were observed only infrequently. The typical children, on the other hand, used communication for a much more varied set of functions, including many more of the social purposes not seen in the children with autism. Similar findings in younger children with autism were reported by Stone, Ousley, Yoder, Hogan, and Hepburn (1997).

Why Do People with Autism Repeat What They Hear?

A proportion of individuals with autism have highly-developed *rote memory* skills for verbal language, enabling them to repeat lengthy segments of language, such as dialogue from videotapes or television commercials, answers to questions, etc. (Dawson, 1996). Others with autism repeat less complex language such as questions, phrases, etc. that have been said to them or said in their presence. This repetition of language is generally referred to as "*echolalia*." Echolalia is often described as either "delayed" or "immediate" depending on the interval (usually hours or days in the case of delayed echolalia) between the language that was heard and its repetition.

Echolalia used to be considered by some to be a symptom to overcome through behavior management (Lovaas, 1977). However, groundbreaking research by Prizant and colleagues (Prizant & Duchan, 1981; Prizant & Rydell, 1984; Rydell & Mirenda, 1994) demonstrated that echolalia is often used by youngsters with autism communicatively and for a variety of purposes, including turn-taking, planning or "rehearsing" behavior, answering questions, and communicating "yes." It is now generally recognized that echolalia can serve communicative functions, but it may also lead observers to overestimate both the receptive understanding and pragmatic skills of those individuals (Twachtman-Cullen, 2000; Wetherby et al., 1997), since the echoed language is generally at a more advanced level than the expressive language that the individual can generate spontaneously (Prizant & Rydell, 1984).

Are There Alternatives to Spoken Language?

Because individuals with autism tend to have relatively stronger visual than auditory skills (Boucher & Lewis, 1989; Hermelin & O'Connor, 1970; Schuler & Baldwin, 1981), a substantial number are able to learn visually-based language better than spoken language. In the 1970's and 80's, there was optimism in the field that *sign language* would be a good option for people with autism (Kiernan, 1983). However, over time it has become clear that there are issues that make sign language a less functional alternative for people with autism than had originally been thought. Mirenda and Erickson (2000) refer to these issues as "the three I's": imitation, iconicity, and intelligibility. By this they mean that functional use of sign language appears to require a foundation of good imitation skills (often deficient in children with autism), that some signs do not have an obvious relationship with the concept they convey, rendering them as symbolic (that is, non-iconic) as verbal language, and that well-developed motor coordination and motor planning skills are required for signs to be clear and comprehensible (Seal & Bonvillian, 1997) in addition to the fact that most potential communication partners do not know sign language (intelligibility). Further, the attention problems of people with autism can make it difficult to notice and focus on the sign before it is finished and gone (Layton & Watson, 1995).

Other forms of visual language are *pictorial* and *written* language, which can be used to augment both receptive understanding and expressive communication on the part of individuals with autism (Bondy & Frost, 2001; Mirenda, 2001; Mirenda & Erickson, 2000). Many individuals with autism are able to gain some meaning from written language, although another phenomenon occasionally seen is "hyperlexia," which refers to the ability to decode written words without associated comprehension (Nation, 1999). Mirenda and Erickson (2000) described the characteristics of hyperlexia as "1) word reading skills that exceed what is predicted or expected based on cognitive and language abilities; 2) compulsive or indiscriminate reading of words; 3) onset of ability when the child is 2–5 years old; and 4) onset of ability in the absence of direct instruction" (pp. 349–350).

Hyperlexia, like echolalic speech, can potentially mislead observers into overestimating the person's functional abilities; however, it remains true that written language can provide meaningful information to some individuals with autism. Mirenda and Erickson (2000) summarized the results of a model demonstration project that found that exposing young children with autism to "literacy artifacts" such as books, markers, magnetic letters, etc., and encouraging literacy-related activities, resulted in "measurable growth in emergent reading and writing skills" during a 3-month period (pp. 353–354). In an exploratory study with adolescents, Schairer and Nelson (1996) demonstrated that for some individuals, elements of written conversations were longer, more complex, more focused, and more spontaneous than in oral conversations.

Even if written words do not become meaningful, it is possible to teach many people with autism to associate meaning with less abstract, more iconic visual information, such as line drawings, photographs, and product labels (such as the "golden arches" of McDonalds). With this foundation, teachers and families can supplement or replace verbal directions with pictorial or written schedules, reminders, and directions that can make even complex tasks understandable to people with autism (Hodgdon, 1999; Janzen, 2003; Krantz, MacDuff, & McClannahan, 1993; MacDuff, Krantz, & McClannahan, 1993; Peterson, Bondy, Vincent, & Finnegan, 1995, Stiebel, 1999; see also Chapter 4, Structured Teaching). Further, even individuals who have both autism and significant mental retardation have the potential to learn a basic communicative exchange process using objects or pictures for the purpose of requesting what they want (Frost & Bondy, 1994; Lancioni, 1983; Layton & Watson, 1995; Schwartz, Garfinkle, & Bauer, 1998).

Does Using Alternative Communication Interfere with Speech Development?

Some families resist the use of alternative forms of communication because of concerns that these would impede the development of speech. However, there is some evidence that nonverbal autistic children who have been taught either sign language or a picture exchange communication system eventually begin speaking too (Konstantareas, 1996; Magiati & Howlin, 2003). For example, Frost and Bondy (1994) reported that 44 of 66 preschool children who had used the Picture Exchange Communication System (PECS) for a year began speaking independently, and 14 others developed some speech. Speech generally began after the children were using between 30 and 100 pictures to communicate various wishes. Barrera, Lobato-Barrera and Sulzer-Azaroff (1980) found that a nonverbal $4\frac{1}{2}$ child learned and used words best through the combination of sign language and oral language simultaneously (that is "total communication") compared to either modality separately. Yoder and Layton (1988) and Layton (1988) described an experiment comparing various combinations of speech and signs (speech alone, signs alone, simultaneous communication, alternating speech and sign) with 60 "minimally verbal" children with autism (average age around 5 years). They found that all methods were equally effective in eliciting speech production and spontaneous language for children who had good verbal imitation skills. For children with poor verbal imitation skills, speech alone was the *least* effective method of stimulating spontaneous use of speech; the other methods were not significantly different from each other. Lord (2000) concluded that "there is no evidence that . . . alternative method such as pictures or sign language or gestures, slow down progress as long as everyone keeps talking as well." (p. 266).

Summary of Communication and Language Development in Autism

Communication is the broad category of behaviors that intentionally convey information from one person to another, while language is the sub-category of communication that uses an abstract symbol system. The development of communication skills is important for many reasons, among them social, emotional, and behavioral. If youngsters with autism can learn the spoken and written versions of their native language, these goals are certainly the optimal focus for communication interventions. Unfortunately, however, because of the multiple, lifelong cognitive deficits and disorders associated with autism, most individuals are not able to master normal language skills.

Various factors appear to interfere with the development of expressive communication and language skills in autism. These factors can include limited comprehension, lack of social-communicative intent, generalized difficulty with initiating behavior, specific auditory processing deficits, and/or mental retardation.

A substantial proportion of people with autism do not develop useful speech. Another segment develops some speech, including the use of typical sounds and grammatical structures of their language, but usually with disorders of prosody in connected speech and difficulty with word meaning. Some individuals memorize and repeat segments of verbal language (echolalia). Echolalia can have some communicative functions, but it is not equivalent to spontaneous expressive language, and may lead observers to an inflated estimate of both expressive and receptive skills. The most universally disordered aspect of autistic language is pragmatics, which is the meaningful use of language in a social context.

Because of the relatively stronger visual-perceptual skills of individuals with ASD, communication systems with a visual component are often more meaningful and effective than verbal language. Sign language has been of only limited utility because it is often as abstract and transient as verbal language. However, communication systems that involve pictures, photographs, and/or written words have generally been found to be very useful, both for receptive understanding and expressive use. Even some people with autism who do not speak much are able to read with a certain degree of comprehension. Only through trial and observation can it be determined whether written material is useful in a particular situation for a particular individual. The use of alternative communication systems appears to support, rather than interfere with, the development of verbal language.

RESEARCH LITERATURE ON COMMUNICATION AND LANGUAGE INTERVENTIONS IN AUTISM

Although there is general agreement in the field about the observable characteristics of the communication and language of individuals with ASD, there is more controversy about teaching and intervention techniques (see Konstanta-reas, 1996; Prizant & Wetherby, 1998; and Wetherby, Prizant, & Schuler, 2000 for discussions of these issues). Most psycholinguistic researchers in the area of autism, however, agree with the following principles.

1. Language interventions must be individualized; there is no language curriculum that fits all youngsters (Koegel, Koegel, Frea, & Smith, 1995; Layton & Watson, 1995; Twachtman-Cullen, 1995; Wetherby et al., 1997).

2. Language develops best through the technique of 'scaffolding,' which is the process of connecting the new elements to be learned onto old elements already mastered. For example, in linguistic scaffolding known words are needed in new situations, new functions are taught for existing words, new meanings of words are introduced in familiar contexts, etc. (Klinger & Dawson, 1992; Watson, Lord, Schaffer, & Schopler, 1989).

Janzen (2003) discussed in detail how to build on a student's existing knowledge to approach teach abstract language concepts, including using multiple concrete "positive" examples of the concept *and* "negative" examples that demonstrate what the concept is not (for example, to teach 'red' use red apples and red trucks, but also green apples and yellow trucks). She also described methods for expanding the meaning of the concept and preventing learned errors during instruction.

3. Modern psycholinguistic theory also holds that using words functionally rests on a foundation of preverbal social-communication skills. In other words, learning language is not equivalent to learning to say words; rather, "the development of preverbal communication is a necessary precursor to the development of the intentional use of language to communicate. Words should be mapped onto preverbal communication skills" (Wetherby et al., 1997, p. 515).

There are several key preverbal skills and conditions that form the basis for communication and language development (Layton & Watson, 1995). Most basic is *something to communicate about.* People first learn to understand and communicate about objects, activities, or experiences that are meaningful to them. Therefore, individuals with autism need to have the understanding that there is predictable order in the world rather than random chaos, and that desirable objects and activities have "names" (even if these are non-linguistic) that can be understood receptively and used expressively. (See Janzen, 2003 and Chapter 4, Structured Teaching in this book for techniques for providing meaningful structure and organization to the environment). Typically developing children first learn to understand the language "names" related to desired food, drink, and toys, enjoyable activities (such as "outside" or "go in the car") and social interactions (names of people, words for social games like "pattycake;" Lord & Paul, 1997). Children with ASD also first learn to understand and use communication related to things that are of interest to them. The interests of youngsters with autism might be atypical (for example, sifting beans, eating ice chips, or watching the weather channel), but the general principle remains that they will learn first to understand about topics of interest to them.

Further, the *responsiveness of caregivers* is an important influence on the development of communication skills. Siller and Sigman (2002) recently reported results indicating that the ability of a sample of mothers to "synchronize" their comments in an undemanding way with their child's focus of interest at the time was significantly related to the child's eventual expressive language development. (Watson [1998] had earlier reported that mothers of preschool children with autism commented on their child's focus of interest as much as mothers of typically developing children of the same age.)

Another preverbal foundation for expressive communication is an *understanding of cause and effect.* Although most youngsters with autism develop this understanding well in terms of the physical world (for example, learning to manipulate toys and other objects to get a certain effect, learning to open doors, etc.), they are less likely to understand that they can have an effect on people. Part of teaching communication, therefore, will involve teaching that movements and/or vocalizations lead to predictable, desirable reactions on the part of people. Understanding this cause and effect forms the basis for *communicative intent*, which is the very basic motivation to use signals in order to have an effect on another person (Prizant & Wetherby, 1987). Although this motivation develops smoothly in typical children, often it must be explicitly stimulated in children with autism (Wetherby, 1986).

In order to be an active communicator rather than a passive recipient of others' communication, the child with autism must have a way to express himself/herself. So a further prerequisite for expressive communication is a *clear communicative behavior* that is associated with the object, activity, or experience the individual wants to communicate about, and that is understood by the receiver. Spoken words are the most typical and most efficient communication behavior, but there are multiple other options for individuals who cannot master spoken language. These range from vocalizing sounds or using simple gestures (such as eye gaze and/or pointing), to touching or handing objects, pictures or words to another person, to advanced skills of signing, writing, or typing.

There is also evidence that some ability to *imitate* is a prerequisite for developing communication and language skills (Carr, Pridal, & Dores, 1984; Curcio, 1978; Lord, 2000; Miranda & Erickson, 2000). Klinger and Dawson (1992) have described methods for stimulating imitation skills, beginning with imitation *of* the child with autism, then progressing to delayed imitation, turn-taking, introduction of different movements for the *child* to imitate, and stimulation of eye contact. Similar themes are found in the work of Greenspan and Wieder (2000).

4. Many expressive communication skills must be explicitly taught, even for verbal children.

At early developmental levels, this might take the form of teaching the student to hand an object or picture to someone (e.g., PECS system; Bondy & Frost, 2001). For students learning to use words in some form, Prizant, Schuler, Wetherby, and Rydell (1997) provide an elegant list of selection criteria for vocabulary to teach (including words for desired objects; words to replace socially unacceptable behavior [such as "no" instead of screaming]; words for early concepts like "all gone" and "mine;" and names of significant people). Working with more advanced youngsters, Koegel and colleagues (Koegel, 1995; Koegel, Camarata, Valdez-Menchaca, & Koegel, 1998) described teaching them to ask various questions, including "what's that?" and "whose is it?" Similarly, Krantz and McClannahan (1998) described using very simple written 'scripts' to teach three preschool children to say "watch me" or "look" while playing with toys. Sarokoff, Taylor, and Poulson (2001) used written scripts with school-age children with autism to teach them to make conversational comments about various objects and games they were involved with. McGee, Krantz and McClannahan (1984) taught adolescents specific phrases to use to express enjoyment of games (such as "great play") and to stand up for themselves (such as "it's my turn now"). Charlop and Milstein (1989) demonstrated that watching videotaped models of conversation was effective in increasing various aspects of conversational speech for three adolescents. Additional studies involving verbal scripts for social interactions are reviewed in Goldstein (2002).

5. It is important to set up situations that stimulate communication.

There is some degree of paradox or contradiction in the goal of "teaching spontaneous communication," since by definition spontaneity is unpredictable and not under external control (Hubbell, 1977). However, teachers, therapists, and families can arrange situations in which spontaneous communication is more likely to occur (Twachtman-Cullen, 1995). In general, the technique of establishing then violating routines and expectations is seen as a useful stimulus for communication (Klinger and Dawson, 1992; Janzen, 2003; Rollins, Wambacq, Dowell, Mathews, & Reese, 1998; Schuler, Prizant, & Wetherby, 1997). At early developmental levels, this can take the form of playing a simple movement/sound game with the child or imitating the child's behavior, then delaying the game or imitation to give the child the opportunity to indicate that he wants the adult to continue or respond (Aldred, Pollard, & Adams, 2001). For students with more advanced language skills, one strategy is the establishment of "Joint Action Routines" (Snyder-McLean, Solomonson, McLean, & Sack, 1984). These authors define such a routine as "a ritualized interaction pattern, involving joint action, unified by a specific theme or goal, which follows a logical sequence, including a clear beginning point, and in which each participant plays a recognized role, with specific response expectancies, that is essential to the successful completion of that sequence" (p. 214). In other words, these are meaningful sequences of social-communicative interactions; examples are playing store, preparing a snack with a group, or acting out a story (such as Little Red Riding Hood). By engaging repeatedly in such Joint Action Routines, children can come to anticipate and initiate the words and phrases involved; furthermore, variations and surprises introduced by the teacher or by another child can stimulate spontaneous communication.

Related techniques that have been found to evoke spontaneous communication are *using familiar objects in unusual ways,* such as using spoons to 'comb' hair; using a backpack as a cushion; putting shoes on hands instead of feet, and *'sabotaging'* familiar materials, such as removing puzzle pieces; putting desired objects into see-through containers that the child cannot open; or putting snack items on a high shelf (Layton & Watson, 1995; McClenny, Roberts, & Layton, 1992).

6. The ultimate communication skill is spontaneous initiation of communication. Youngsters with autism (and other developmental disabilities) are at risk of becoming passive, prompt-dependent communicators unless care is taken to support and encourage spontaneity (Hubbell, 1977; Prizant, Wetherby, & Rydell, 2000; Twachtman-Cullen, 1995). To counteract this risk, it is important to

- Leave the youngster enough time to formulate and initiate a communication (Layton & Watson, 1995; Rydell & Mirenda, 1994)
- Follow the child's lead in determining topics of communication
- Minimize yes/no questions (Capps et al., 1998)
- Use natural reinforcers/consequences rather than artificial or unrelated ones (such as giving a child a piece of candy for labeling a picture of a banana)
- Reinforce all communication attempts

Such techniques are variously referred to as "natural language paradigm" (Koegel, Koegel, & Carter, 1998), "milieu teaching" (Koegel, 1995), "incidental teaching" (McGee, Morrier, & Daly, 1999), the Developmental Social-Pragmatic Model (Prizant et al., 2000), or a "facilitative" (rather than "directive") style (Mirenda & Donnellen, 1986).

PRINCIPLES OF THE TEACCH APPROACH TO COMMUNICATION AND LANGUAGE SKILLS

The TEACCH Structured Teaching approach to communication incorporates the major principles highlighted by modern psycholinguistic research.

Individualization

We recognize that the communication/language program for each individual must be unique. While some strategies and goals are generally helpful, the particular areas of understanding, confusion, and emerging skill are different for each individual. There is no standard TEACCH language curriculum because there is no sequence or content of skills that is appropriate for all students.

Scaffolding

The principle of scaffolding is deeply ingrained in the TEACCH approach to teaching all new skills, including communication/language skills. We have long recognized that introducing or changing too many variables at the same time is ineffective at best, and at worst overwhelming for people with ASD. For example, rather than going to a new place to play a new game with a new person, the TEACCH approach would be to keep two of those elements familiar, while introducing one new element; for example, the student might go to a new place to play a familiar game with familiar companions. Thus, what has already been learned or experienced becomes the scaffold on which new learning is built.

Five basic elements of communication that form the scaffold have been described by Watson et al. (1989):

1. The specific *word* or phrase used (or the meaning of the communication, if it is not in the form of a word)
2. The *form* of the communication (such as a motor movement, gesture, vocalization, picture, sign(s), written word, spoken word(s)
3. The *function* of the communication (such as requesting, getting attention, rejecting or refusing, commenting, giving information, seeking information, expressing feelings, or participating in a social routine)
4. The *context* of the communication (such as with teachers/parents, with other familiar children, with familiar adults, with other adults, with other children, in groups, during meals, during free time, etc.)
5. The *semantic category* of the communication (such as object wanted, action being done, location of a person, etc.)

Examples of a scaffolding approach to choosing communication goals, therefore, would be

- Teaching the child to say "bathroom" instead of saying "pee pee" (that is, teaching a new word)
- Teaching the child to hand a teacher a picture of a bathroom rather than saying "buh-buh" (that is, changing the form of the communication)
- Teaching a child to say "bathroom" before he is permitted to go into the bathroom, instead of when he is in the bathroom looking around (that is, changing the function from labeling to requesting)
- Teaching the child to say "bathroom" to other teachers and school personnel, instead of only to his teacher (that is, changing the context in which he asked to use the bathroom)
- Teaching the child to say "where bathroom?" instead of just bathroom (that is, changing the semantic category from an object to include the concept of location)

The optimal outcome is large, flexible pool of spontaneous utterances that are functional in a range of everyday situations. Selecting the particular goals to be worked on must be based on careful observation of the student's current communication skills and patterns (that is, the scaffold). It is also important for the teaching program to be balanced in terms of expanding vocabulary, functions, contexts, and semantic categories (and also forms, for those students whose use of spoken words is limited). For example, teaching only vocabulary, or only the function of labeling, or communication only in the classroom, or only in response to direct questions, is unbalanced and not very functional.

Foundation of Preverbal Communication Skills

Many aspects of the TEACCH approach serve the function of providing the individual with something to communicate about. Understanding that there is meaning and predictability in the environment is fundamental for communicating about that environment. If food appears at random times and places, if the individual is pulled from location to location without knowing where he is going, if objects are presented and withdrawn unpredictably, the person with autism is unlikely to learn concepts such as "snack," "dining room," "go outside," "time to play," or "work is finished." The TEACCH Structured Teaching approach means arranging the environment so that the individual knows where to be, what to do, how long to do it, and what will happen next (see Chapter 4, Structured Teaching). Structure enables the person to understand where he is in the physical environment, to focus attention on meaningful objects and people, and to engage in activities in a predictable sequence. This organizes the individual's world sufficiently for him to learn to attach receptive and labels and expressive labels to meaningful aspects of his world.

In the TEACCH approach, developing the understanding that interactions with people are pleasurable, meaningful, and effective is also important. One-to-one teaching sessions, structured and unstructured play times, and meals are among the settings in which the individual learns that caregivers are responsive, interested, willing to provide verbal labels for items or activities of special interest to the person, and willing to respond to emerging attempts at both requesting and social communication.

Clear Communication Behavior

Another goal of our communication program is that the communicative act be easily understood by the person receiving it, and ideally by as many people as possible. Often parents and teachers may come to recognize and understand even atypical communicative acts like very subtle movements, nonsense words, or idiosyncratic echoed phrases that are used communicatively (such as when a child repeated a line from a commercial, "tired eyes, aching feet" when his eyes were stinging from chlorine in a swimming pool, and he wanted eye drops). However, if students can be taught to use forms of communication that are more understandable to their community in general, such as spoken or written words, line drawings, or photographs, they will have a much higher degree of control and independence in their lives.

Teaching Specific Words/Structures

Practices within the TEACCH program are consistent with the approach of teaching and stimulating specific words and phrases. We begin with an emphasis on receptive understanding linked to expressive use. For students with significant mental retardation, the 'words' often take the form of objects, pictures, or other concrete and minimally symbolic materials. For more advanced students, formal language structures (such as nouns, verbs, adjectives, prepositions, etc.) are taught both receptively and expressively. Specifics of TEACCH procedures are discussed in more detail in the following sections.

An Environment that Stimulates Communication

In the TEACCH Structured Teaching approach, structure is a means to an end, rather than an end in itself. That is, structure is not in place in order to control the student's behavior and suppress his/her spontaneity; rather, it is used to make the student's environment understandable and predictable, so that spontaneous communication can emerge. A typical Structured Teaching program includes substantial one-to-one attention, using objects and activities that are of interest to the student, and incorporating multiple opportunities for the student to make choices. Thus, Structured Teaching is very compatible with the "facilitative" style (Mirenda & Donnellan, 1986) or "natural language paradigm" (Koegel, 1995).

Meaningful Spontaneous Communication

The goal of the TEACCH approach for all people with autism is *meaningful, spontaneous communication.* We can know that a particular communication is meaningful to the person with autism if he or she uses it spontaneously (Watson et al., 1989). This means that the person initiates and carries out the communicative act without being prompted, questioned, guided, assisted, etc. Although *learning* communication skills often requires some of those supports, only the communicative acts that people use spontaneously let us know that the communication is truly meaningful and useful to them.

Some traditional speech/language and behavioral therapies have focused on teaching vocabulary and other aspects of language in artificial settings, such as sitting at a table labeling pictures or answering questions about them. Some children with autism are 'successful' in these drills, because of their strong rote memories and ability to learn to respond compliantly to directions. However, these techniques do not address the more fundamental goal of spontaneous communication of personal desires and ideas. For example, many verbal children with autism can learn to label a picture of a "zipper" and yet, if they are cold on the playground, be unable to approach a teacher and ask for their zipper to be closed. In this scenario, the communication 'skill' learned in a treatment session was not truly functional (Landa, 2000; Prizant & Wetherby, 1998). In the TEACCH approach, on the other hand, communication goals focus on learning and using meaningful labels/words/phrases in real-life situations.

TEACCH APPROACH TO COMMUNICATION
SKILLS FOR NONVERBAL AND
LOW-VERBAL INDIVIDUALS

For students at beginning stages of associating labels with meaningful materials and activities in their day, we begin by using consistent concrete objects. Students with somewhat more developed cognitive skills may learn to associate pictures or other two-dimensional representations. Some students with very limited verbal language skills are nevertheless able to understand written encoding of language (that is, recognize written words).

Objects

The most basic and concrete form of communication uses the actual objects that are part of the activity being communicated about. This requires the least symbolic reasoning, and is therefore the simplest for individuals with significant mental retardation and autism to learn. Examples are:

- A spoon or cup for mealtimes
- A roll of toilet paper for going to the bathroom
- A ball, plastic shovel, or other toy for going outside to play
- A backpack for going home
- A different item for going outside for a walk (such as a "belly bag" that has something in it that is used on the walk, such as chalk to mark on the sidewalk, or bread scraps to throw for birds)
- A wash cloth for taking a bath
- A pajama top for going to bed

As described previously, teaching this system begins with helping the student to associate the object with the activity. Therefore, the *same* object should be given or shown to the student before the activity *each time* it takes place. For very young or low functioning students, the object can be handed to them. Students at a somewhat higher level can be taken to a consistent location in the home or classroom where the communicative object is located. Sometimes we build a special shelf in a convenient location, then direct the student there at each transition between activities. With repetition, children learn the routine of going to the transition place to find an object that lets them know what is going to happen next. As discussed earlier, having this information can reduce the confusion and disorganization that people with autism often experience. It is very important that the student learn to go to the transition area *independently*, then to proceed to the activity *independently*. The student might at first need gestures or mild physical guidance to go through this process, but these should be faded as soon as possible, because the goal of all aspects of the TEACCH approach is as much independence as possible (see Chapter 4, Structured Teaching).

Next steps in the understanding of objects include learning to associate smaller, more *symbolic objects* with activities (such as a toy car or bus for going home), which can be more portable and practical than the actual objects used in the activity, and learning to understand a *series of objects* that communicate the next several activities (for example, work then outside then wash hands). In the latter scenario, the student would continue going to the transition area to take one object, but would see the other objects representing later activities, and in this way be exposed to information about upcoming events. (See Chapter 4, Structured Teaching for further discussion of the use of visually-based schedules.)

Understanding object-based communication can be a foundation for the development of object-based *expressive* communication. For example, once students have developed firm associations between specific objects and events, they can learn to make simple choices by reaching for the object that is part of the activity they prefer. Some students can choose among a large number of objects, and can learn to hand the communicative object to a caregiver. For individuals at this level, it is important to keep the schedule and the choice board physically separate and visually distinct, so that these individuals are not confused about available choices.

Line Drawings

Simple line drawings can be used in the same way as objects. A single picture is handed to the student before each activity. The student carries the picture to the location where the activity takes place, and puts it in a receptacle (such as a small basket, envelope, or library card pocket) that has a matching picture on it. (The purpose of this is to help the student stay focused on his destination as he goes there.)

As with objects, the receptive communication system using line drawings begins by handing the student the picture. Eventually most students can handle a double transition of first being directed to a transition area where one picture is waiting, then following the picture to the location of designated activity. The system can then usually be advanced to a series of pictures, at first for several activities, then in many cases for the entire period of the day that the individual will be using that schedule (such as the school day, or workday, afternoon until bedtime, etc.).

Expressively, once students have learned to associate the pictures with the objects and activities, they can use pictures to make choices and indicate their wishes. For example, this could include pictures of

- Specific foods (pictures from magazines or food packages might be useful)
- Specific toy or materials
- Activities such as going outside, playing with water, going bowling, etc.

Some teachers, parents, and others in the individual's circle might be able to draw simple pictures that can be used for communication. Several excellent computer graphics programs are also available commercially or on the internet that allow the user to vary the size of the drawing, to print it with or without a written word below it, and to select from a large variety of drawings to represent the concept. Drawings can be colored if this seems to aide the person's interest or understanding. Sources of pictures include the Boardmaker software program (available from the Autism Society of North Carolina, (919) 743-0204 or *www.autismsociety-nc.org)* or the following websites: *www.do2learn.com, www.kidaccess.com.*

Photographs/Pictures

Photographs can be taken of various elements of the person's environment, or pictures from magazines can be used. The system of using photographs or pictures is the same as that with line drawing. All options may need to be tried, because some individuals have difficulty understanding the meaning of drawings, but can understand life-like photographs. For others, the opposite is true: line drawings appear to be clearer and more meaningful, while photographs are too cluttered to convey information clearly. Also, some individuals with ASD take photographs too literally, and assume that the situation they are going to will be *exactly* like the picture. Then, for example, when the specific food item in the "lunch" picture is not served, they become distressed. We have found it helpful to have a Polaroid or digital camera available, to take pictures of specific toys, people, foods, etc. and to modify them as needed so that the individual using them system finds them clear, meaningful, and adequate for independent functioning.

Written Words

Students with ASD are very visually-oriented and generally have a profile of scattered cognitive skills, with marked strengths and weaknesses. Some students begin at very young ages to notice written words if they are available, and to associate them with meaning. *Just because a person with autism does not talk, it cannot be assumed that he or she does not have some level of reading comprehension.* As with many other aspects of these students' skills, this can be determined only through observation on the part of family members and teachers. Even if the student's functional receptive communication in a classroom or at home is very limited at first, and a system of line drawings or photographs is what they need to function independently, these can be paired with written words and additional exercises can be done to help students make the associations, so that eventually it might be possible to 'fade' the pictures/photographs (that is, gradually reduce their size or content) while the written words remain.

The selection of which visual communication system to use must be individualized. *If all students in a classroom or other setting are using the same communication system, it is likely that there is insufficient individualization.* Several systems may need to be tried, to determine which is most meaningful to the student. As a general rule, lower functioning students have difficulty with anything other than objects. Students who generally function at a high level (and any others who have been observed to be interested in letters) should probably be exposed to written words, in addition to pictures or photographs. Determining which individuals will respond better to line drawings, magazine pictures, or photographs can be done only through observation and trial and error.

As described above, the principle of scaffolding is important within the TEACCH approach. Next steps involved building on the skills and understanding the student has, to add more words, semantic categories (that is, naming objects, naming actions, describing locations), functions, and contexts. In addition, we work to help each student achieve the highest developmental level possible, in terms of communication forms (that is, object, pictures, spoken words, typing, etc.)

TEACCH APPROACH TO LANGUAGE SKILLS
FOR VERBAL INDIVIDUALS WITH ASD

For those students who have mastered the foundation-level skills for communication and who use verbal language, either spontaneously or in imitation, standard speech and language therapy goals are appropriate. That is, these youngsters can work on goals such as expanding vocabulary (receptive and expressive), expanding the length and type of phrases/sentences used, correct use of plurals, verb tenses, pronouns, etc. Typical techniques of modeling, prompting, reinforcing, and setting up situations to stimulate language are used.

There are some language problems specific to autism that call for specialized goals and strategies (Twachtman, 1995; Prizant et al., 1997). Verbal students with autism have difficulty using their language to meet their social needs and promote their interactions with others. Specifically, problems typically include poor conversational skills and may also include persistent questioning or long monologues. TEACCH approaches these difficulties by using students' strengths in visual skills and in learning specific rules to teach them social-linguistic rules and expectations that may be too subtle for them to infer independently. As always, these general principles must be individualized in creative, even unorthodox ways for each student.

Conversational Skills

Typical problems with conversations include identifying topics for conversation, taking turns to maintain the conversational flow, and staying on the topic.

Identifying Topics for Conversation

There are several reasons why individuals with ASD have difficulty related to topics of conversations. People with autism often like to talk about their specialized interests, rather than about topics of more general interest to others. Related to this, they may have difficulty recognizing what topics actually are of interest to their peers, family members, and others. Further, during conversations they can become so focused on what they want to talk about that they don't attend to the other person or respond to what the person is saying.

TEACCH strategies designed to help students with ASD with these topic identification and maintenance problems have several components. We typically start with activities that assist our students in identifying topics of general interest for conversations. One way to do this is to have a group, including non-handicapped peers and/or teachers, list topics they like to talk about and put each topic in a hat. The topics are then drawn from the hat, one at a time, and placed in the center of the table. The group has a brief conversation on each topic; if any students with ASD deviate from the topic, a visual cue redirecting them back to the paper on the table is usually sufficient to get them back on task.

In order to help students remember these appropriate topics of conversation, homework assignments can be helpful, particularly for adolescents. For homework, each student is assigned one of the topics from the day's discussion and required to call three peers for a brief discussion on that topic. This assignment is generally effective and well-received because many students with ASD see family members get frequent phone calls but often receive none themselves. Using this technique, they are actively involved in communicating on the telephone in the evening, just as other members of the family frequently do. Parents generally like these assignments also because it makes them feel good that their youngsters can participate in this normal evening adolescent activity.

For students who have difficulty identifying what topic everyone is talking about, we have sometimes taught a way of introducing a conversation so that the topic under discussion is perfectly clear to everyone. These students are encouraged to start a conversation by saying, "I am interested in talking about _____. Are you interested in talking about that?" If the other person says, "Yes," then the person with ASD is encouraged to continue. If the person says, "No," then the person with ASD asks, "What are you interested in talking about?" and then is instructed to proceed from there with the other person's topic.

Taking Turns in Conversation

For conversational problems that occur because people with ASD have difficulty with the back-and-forth of reciprocal conversations, a visual cue can be a helpful reminder of whose turn it is to talk. One visual cue that has been very popular among our students is a microphone. The person holding the microphone is the one who has the floor to talk and others must wait until it is passed to them before starting their part of the conversation. If someone talks without the microphone, a visual cue of pointing to the microphone is generally all that is needed to remind everyone who should be speaking.

Once basic conversational turn-taking is mastered, several additional strategies can be effective for maintaining the flow of conversations. For some individuals with ASD, visual cues and checklists can be helpful. For example, once the topic of conversation is established, you might write a reminder that this student is to say three things about the topic. As he says each one, he makes a mark indicating that one is completed. When he has made his three statements (and three marks) as part of an ongoing conversation, that is his cue that the conversation should end. This can be especially helpful for students who tend to go on and on and don't know when to end conversations. For more advanced individuals, it may helpful to be explicit that it is time to end the conversation (for example, "I enjoyed talking with you. I have to go now. Goodbye [or See you later])."

Another strategy that can be helpful is to teach the individual with ASD to respond to questions and then ask the same questions back to the questioner. For example, if he is asked what he had for lunch on a given day, he might respond saying a hamburger and a drink, and then ask his questioner what he had for lunch. This can be an effective conversational strategy because many people ask questions of students with ASD, which provides many opportunities for the student to reciprocate. Further, the behavior that the individual with ASD is supposed to demonstrate (answering the question then asking the same question in return) is clear and relatively simple.

Staying on Topic

Once topics are identified and turn-taking has been learned, the next skill is staying on a topic and maintaining a conversation with another person. Teaching question-asking can be a helpful way to teach an individual with ASD to direct the conversation to another person and maintain the topic. Obviously this strategy is neither necessary nor desirable if the person with ASD is a perseverative questioner (see the following section). For others, however, this technique can be a helpful way of maintaining everyone's focus on a specific topic. For example, it can be effective to encourage the student with ASD to ask questions about his immediate situation. If he is in a restaurant, he might ask the other person if he likes this restaurant, if he has been here before, and what he has done since the last time that he was in the restaurant. This can also be done for a town, school, hotel, store, and a wide variety of places where the person with ASD might find himself engaged in a spontaneous conversation.

Sometimes topics can be identified and turn-taking established, but still the person with ASD has difficulty with the conversation, because the topics that are of general interest to other people are things the individual with ASD knows nothing about. In this case, it is helpful to select topics that are based on experiences that the members of the group have shared. Some examples would be a field trip to a fun place, an assembly around an interesting activity, or a recent movie. Alternatively, the teacher or group leader might consider bringing in a short video tape for everyone to observe and discuss. Watching a short video about a topic of general interest, or bringing something to demonstrate to the group might provide a direct experience that everyone would enjoy talking about.

Other Issues

Very advanced students may also benefit from individualized Social Stories (Gray, 1998) that deal with their situations and difficulties. For example, these short paragraphs can be used to explain nuances of conversations, such as topics or words that are not appropriate with certain conversational partners or in certain contexts (for example, teasing a boss, talking about personal hygiene a member of the opposite sex, telling jokes at a funeral).

Persistent Questioning

Some verbal youngsters with ASD repeat the same question to the same person with great frequency and persistence. We generally think that this behavior comes from one of two sources: either a desire for social interaction or else confusion about expectations and plans for upcoming events (leading the student to ask, in effect, 'when am I going to do X?' or 'what is going to happen next?'). There are several helpful approaches to reducing this behavior, which parents and others typically find quite annoying.

If the student is using questions as a way of initiating social contact, the most helpful approach is to give him other ways to achieve this same goal. For example, we might provide students with written 'conversation starters' that they can be prompted to use when they appear to be trying to engage someone in a social interaction. In other situations, we might show the student visually that he can ask a finite number of questions, after which he needs to return to his work or other structured activity. Associated with this intervention, we might also show him on his schedule when he will have an opportunity for social time/conversation.

If the student's persistent questioning reflects his confusion about expectations and plans, the most helpful approach is to provide him with concrete, visual information that answers his question. Examples would include:

- A written or pictorial *schedule* of activities for the day
- A *calendar* of the week or the month
- A *written explanation* of the expected sequence of events that is shown or given to the person, who can then refer back to it

For example, if an individual with autism repeatedly asks when he will be going to the swimming pool, his *schedule* might indicate:

- Eat lunch
- Math class
- Swimming pool
- Snack
- Bus

A *calendar* might show the days of the week, with an arrow to indicate the current date and a picture of the swimming pool on the day that the trip to the pool will occur. Each morning the student could assist or observe as the arrow is advanced, so that the student can see that it is getting closer to the day with the pool picture.

A *written explanation* might be:

> "We usually go to the swimming pool on Friday afternoons. It takes a lot of time to go to the pool because it is far away. We have to take a special bus ride, which is expensive. We do not have enough time or money to go to the pool every day. It is a special treat to go to the pool. We are planning to go to the pool on Friday afternoon. If this plan changes, the teacher will tell you."

Monologues

Some individuals talk about their special interest without apparent awareness of whether the listener is bored, irritated, trying to do something else, etc. One TEACCH approach would be to use the individual's visual interests to redirect him to a different activity. Generally this would be done by showing him a written sentence such as "It's time to get back to work," or "I don't have time to listen right now. I can listen to you after____activity (or around X:XX time)," or "Please stop talking and check your schedule." Generally these individuals also would benefit from Social Stories (Gray, 1998) that explain whatever social convention they are unknowingly violating and/or what social cues they can look for (such as limiting conversations during the work day; the person's glancing at the clock).

SUMMARY

Because of the wide range of skill levels and age levels among individuals who share the diagnosis of autism, the issues involved in addressing their communication needs are complex. The TEACCH approach is built on the fundamental principles of individualization, understanding the characteristic skill pattern in ASD (including visual strengths, difficulty with inferring meaning, and difficulty with generalization), and the importance of functional, spontaneous communication.

REFERENCES

Aldred, C., Pollard, C., and Adams, C. (2001). Child'sTalk: For children with autism and pervasive developmental disorders. *International Journal of Language and Communication Disorders, 36* (Suppl.), 469–474.

American Psychiatric Association. (2000). *Diagnostic and statistical manual of mental disorders* (4th *ed., Text Revision)*. Washington, DC: Author.

Anzalone, M.E. & Williams, G.G. (2000). Sensory processing disorders and motor performance in autism spectrum disorders. In A.M. Wetherby & B.M. Prizant (Eds.), *Autism spectrum disorders: A transactional developmental perspective* (pp. 143–166). Baltimore: Paul Brookes.

Asperger, H. (1991). 'Autistic Psychopathy' in childhood. In U. Frith (Ed. & Trans.), *Autism and Asperger syndrome* (pp. 37–92). Cambridge: Cambridge University Press. (Original work published 1944).

Ballaban-Gil, K., Rapin, I., Tuchman, R., & Shinnar, S. (1996). Longitudinal examination of the behavioral, language, and social changes in a population of adolescents and young adults with autistic disorder. *Pediatric Neurology, 15*, 217–223.

Baltaxe, C.A.M. & Simmons, J.Q. III. (1992). A comparison of language issues in high-functioning autism and related disorders with onset in childhood and adolescence. In E. Schopler & G.B. Mesibov (Eds.), *High functioning individuals with autism* (pp. 201–225). New York: Plenum Press.

Baron-Cohen, S. (1988). Social and pragmatic deficits in autism: Cognitive or affective? *Journal of Autism and Developmental Disorders, 18*, 379–402.

Barrera, R.D., Lobato-Barrera, D., & Sulzer-Azaroff, B. (1980). A simultaneous treatment comparison of three expressive language training programs with a mute autistic child. *Journal of Autism and Developmental Disorders, 10*, 21–37.

Bartolucci, G., Pierce, S.J., & Streiner, D. (1980). Cross-sectional studies of grammatical morphemes in autistic and mentally retarded children. *Journal of Autism and Developmental Disorders, 10*, 39–50.

Bondy, A. & Frost, L. (2001). *A picture's worth: PECS and other visual communication strategies in autism*. Bethesda, MD: Woodbine House.

Bryson, S.E. & Smith, I.M. (1998). Epidemiology of autism: Prevalence, associated characteristics, and implications for research and service delivery. *Mental Retardation and Developmental Disabilities Research Reviews, 4*, 97–103.

Capps, L., Kehres, J., & Sigman, M. (1998). Conversational abilities among children with autism and children with developmental delays. *Autism, 2*, 325–344.

Carr, E.G. & Carlson, J.I. (1993). Reduction of severe behavior problems in the community using a multicomponent treatment approach. *Journal of Applied Behavior Analysis, 26*, 157–172.

Carr, E.G. & Durand, V.M. (1985). Reducing behavior problems through functional communication training. *Journal of Applied Behavior Analysis, 18*, 111–126.

Carr, E.G., Pridal, C., & Dores, P.A. (1984). Speech versus sign comprehension in autistic children: Analysis and prediction. *Journal of Experimental Child psychology, 37*, 587–597.

Charlop, M.H. & Milstein, J.P. (1989). Teaching autistic children conversational speech using video modeling. *Journal of Applied Behavior Analysis, 22*, 275–285.

Curcio, F. (1978). Sensorimotor functioning and communication in mute autistic children. *Journal of Autism and Childhood Schizophrenia, 8*, 281–292.

Davidovitch, M., Glick, L., Holtzman, G., Tirosh, E., & Safir, M.P. (2000). Developmental regression in autism: Maternal perception. *Journal of Autism and Developmental Disorders, 30*, 113–119.

Dawson, G. (1996). Brief Report: Neuropsychology of autism: A report on the state of the science. *Journal of Autism and Developmental Disorders, 26*, 179–184.

Dawson, G. & Watling, R. (2000). Interventions to facilitate auditory, visual, and motor integration in autism: A review of the evidence. *Journal of Autism and Developmental Disorders, 30*, 415–421.

Durand, V.M. & Carr, E.G. (1992). An analysis of maintenance following functional communication training. *Journal of Applied Behavior Analysis, 25*, 777–794.

Eales, M.J. (1993). Pragmatic impairments in adults with childhood diagnoses of autism or developmental receptive language disorder. *Journal of Autism and Developmental Disorders, 23*, 593–617.

Eaves, L.C. & Ho, H.H. (1996). Brief report: Stability and change in cognitive and behavioral characteristics of autism through childhood. *Journal of Autism and Developmental Disorders, 26*, 557–569.

Fine, J., Bartolucci, G., Szatmari, P., & Ginsberg, G. (1994). Cohesive discourse in pervasive developmental disorders. *Journal of Autism and Developmental Disorders, 24*, 315–329.

Frea, W.D. (1995). Social-communicative skills in higher-functioning children with autism. In R.L. Kogel & L.K. Koegel (Eds.), *Teaching children with autism* (pp. 53–66). Baltimore: Paul Brookes.

Frea, W.D., Arnold, C.L., & Vittimberga, G.L. (2001). A demonstration of the effects of augmentative communication on the extreme aggressive behavior of a child with autism within an integrated preschool setting. *Journal of Positive Behavioral Supports, 3*, 194–198.

Frost, L.A. & Bondy, A.S. (1994). *PECS: The picture exchange communication system training manual.* Cherry Hill, NJ: Pyramid Educational Consultants.

Goldberg, W.A., Osnann, K., Filipek, P.A., Laulhere, T., Jarvis, K., Modahl, C. et al. (2003). Language and regression: Assessment and timing. *Journal of Autism and Developmental Disabilities, 33,* 607–616.

Goldstein, H. (2002). Communication intervention for children with autism: A review of treatment efficacy. *Journal of Autism and Developmental Disabilities, 32,* 373–396.

Gray, C. (1998). Social stories and comic strip conversations with students with Asperger syndrome and high-functioning autism. In E. Schopler, G.B. Mesibov, & L.J. Kunce (Eds.), *Asperger syndrome or high-functioning autism?* (pp. 167–198). New York: Plenum Press.

Greenspan, S.I. & Wieder, S. (2000). A developmental approach to difficulties in relating and communicating in autism spectrum disorders and related syndromes. In A.M. Wetherby & B.M. Prizant (Eds.), *Autism spectrum disorders: A transactional developmental perspective* (pp. 279–306). Baltimore: Paul Brookes.

Hermelin, B. & O'Connor, N. (1970). *Psychological experiments with autistic children.* New York: Pergamon Press.

Hodgdon, L. A. (1999). *Solving behavior problems in autism: Improving communication with visual strategies.* Troy, MI: QuirkRoberts.

Hubbell, R. D. (1977). On facilitating spontaneous talking in young children. *Journal of Speech and Hearing Disorders, 42,* 216–231.

Hurtig, R., Ensrud, S., & Tomblin, J.B. (1982). The communicative function of question production in autistic children. *Journal of Autism and Developmental Disorders, 12,* 57–69.

Janzen, J. (2003). *Understanding the nature of autism: A guide to the autism spectrum disorders* (2nd ed.). San Antonio, TX: Therapy Skill Builders.

Kanner, L. (1943). Autistic disturbances of affective contact. *Nervous Child, 2,* 217–250.

Kientz, M.A. & Dunn, W. (1997). A comparison of the performance of children with and without autism on the sensory profile. *The American Journal of Occupational Therapy, 51,* 530–537.

Kiernan, C. (1983). The use on nonvocal communication techniques with autistic individuals. *Journal of Child Psychology and Psychiatry, 3,* 339–375.

Klin, A. & Volkmar, F.R. (1997). Asperger syndrome. In D.J. Cohen & F.R. Volkmar (Eds.), *Handbook of autism and pervasive developmental disorders* (2nd ed.). (pp. 94–122). New York: John Wiley and Sons.

Klinger, L.G. & Dawson, G. (1992). Facilitating early social and communicative development in children with autism. In S. W. Warren & J. Reichle (Eds.), *Causes and effects in communication and language intervention* (pp. 157–186). Baltimore: Paul Brookes.

Koegel, L.K. (1995). Communication and language intervention. In R.L. Koegel & L.K.Koegel (Eds.), *Teaching children with autism* (pp. 17–32). Baltimore: Paul Brookes.

Koegel, L.K. (2000). Interventions to facilitate communication in autism. *Journal of Autism and Developmental Disorders, 30,* 383–391.

Koegel, L.K., Camarata, S.M., Valdez-Menchaca, M., & Koegel, R.L. (1998). Setting generalization of question-asking by children with autism. *American Journal on Mental Retardation, 102,* 346–357.

Koegel, L.K., Koegel, R.L., & Carter, C.M. (1998). Pivotal responses and the natural language teaching paradigm. *Seminars in Speech and Language, 19,* 355–371.

Koegel, L.K., Koegel, R.L. Shoshan, Y., & McNerney, E. (1999). Pivotal response interventions II: Preliminary long-term outcome data. *Journal of the Association for Persons with Severe Handicaps (JASH), 24,* 186–198.

Koegel, R.L., Koegel, L.K., Frea, W.D., & Smith, A.E. (1995). Emerging interventions for children with autism: Longitudinal and lifespan implications. In R.L. Kogel & L.K. Koegel (Eds.), *Teaching children with autism* (pp. 1–15). Baltimore: Paul Brookes.

Konstantareas, M.M. (1996). Communication training approaches in autistic disorder. In J.H. Beitchman, N.J. Cohen, M.M. Konstantareas, & R. Tannock (Eds.), *Language, learning, and behavior disorders* (pp. 467–488). New York: Cambridge University Press.

Konstantareas, M.M. & Beitchman, J.H. (1996). Comorbidity of autistic disorder and specific developmental language disorder: existing evidence and some promising future directions. In

J.H. Beitchman, N.J. Cohen, M.M. Konstantareas, & R. Tannock (Eds.), *Language, learning, and behavior disorders* (pp.178–196). New York: Cambridge University Press.

Krantz, P.J., MacDuff, M.T., & McClannahan, L.E. (1993). Programming participation in family activities for children with autism: Parents' use of photographic activity schedules. *Journal of Applied Behavior Analysis, 26*, 137–138.

Krantz, P.J. & McClannahan, L.E. (1998). Social interaction skills for children with autism: A script-fading procedure for beginning readers. *Journal of Applied Behavior Analysis, 31*, 191–202.

Kurita, H. (1985). Infantile autism with speech loss before the age of thirty months. *Journal of the American Academy of Child Psychiatry, 24*, 191–196.

Kurita, K., Kita, M., & Miyake, Y. (1992). A comparative study of development and symptoms among disintegrative psychosis and infantile autism with and without speech loss. *Journal of Autism and Developmental Disorders, 22*, 175–188.

Lancioni, G. (1983). Using pictorial representations as communication means with low-functioning children. *Journal of Autism and Developmental Disorders, 13*, 87–105.

Landa, R. (2000). Social language use in Asperger syndrome and high-functioning autism. In A. Klin, F.R. Volkmar, & S.S. Sparrow (Eds.), *Asperger syndrome* (pp. 125–155). New York: Guilford.

Layton, T. (1988). Language training with autistic children using four different modes of presentation. *Journal of Communication Disorders, 21*, 333–350.

Layton, T. & Watson, L.R. (1995). Enhancing communication in nonverbal children with autism. In K.A. Quill (Ed.), *Teaching children with autism: Strategies to enhance communication and socialization* (pp. 73–103). New York: Delmar.

Lord, C. (1985). Autism and the comprehension of language. In E. Schopler & G.B. Mesibov (Eds.), *Communication Problems in Autism* (pp. 257–281). New York: Plenum Press.

Lord, C. (2000). Ask the editor. *Journal of Autism and Developmental Disabilities, 30*, 265–266.

Lord, C. & Bailey, A. (2002). Autism spectrum disorders. In M. Rutter & E. Taylor (Eds.), *Child and Adolescent Psychiatry, 4*th edition (pp. 636–663). Malden, MA: Blackwell Science.

Lord, C. & Magill-Evans, J. (1995). Peer interactions of autistic children and adolescents. *Development and Psychopathology, 7*, 611–626.

Lord, C. & Paul, R. (1997). Language and communication in autism. In D.J. Cohen & F.R. Volkmar (Eds.), *Handbook of autism and pervasive developmental disorders* (2nd ed.). (pp. 195–225). New York: John Wiley and Sons.

Lord, C. & Risi, S. (2000). Diagnosis of autism spectrum disorders in young children. In A.M. Wetherby & B.M. Prizant (Eds.), *Autism spectrum disorders: A transactional developmental perspective* (pp. 11–30). Baltimore: Paul Brookes.

Lotter, V. (1966). Epidemiology of autistic conditions in young children. *Social Psychiatry, 1*, 124–137.

Lovaas, O. I. (1977). *The autistic child: Language development through behavior modification*. New York: Irvington.

MacDuff, G.S., Krantz, P.J., & McClannahan, L.E. (1993). Teaching children with autism to use photographic activity schedules: Maintenance and generalization of complex response chains. *Journal of Applied Behavior Analysis, 26*, 89–97.

Magiati, I. & Howlin, P. (2003). A pilot evaluation study of the Picture Exchange Communication System (PECS) for children with autistic spectrum disorders. *Autism, 7*, 297–320.

Mantovani, J.F. (2000). Seizures, Landau-Kleffner syndrome, and autistic regression: Differential diagnosis and treatment. In P.J. Accardo, C. Magnusen, & A.J. Capute (Eds.), *Autism: Clinical and research issues* (pp. 225–240). Baltimore: York Press.

McClenny, C.S., Roberts, J.E., & Layton, T.L. (1992). Unexpected events and their effect on children's language. *Child Language Teaching and Therapy, 8*, 229–245.

McGee, G.G., Krantz, P.J., & McClannahan, L.E. (1984). Conversational skills for autistic adolescents: Teaching assertiveness in naturalistic game settings. *Journal of Autism and Developmental Disorders, 14*, 319–330.

McGee, G.G., Morrier, M.J., & Daly, T. (1999). An incidental teaching approach to early intervention for toddlers with autism. *Journal of the Association for Persons with Severe Handicaps (JASH), 24*, 133–146.

McHale, S.M., Simeonsson, R.J., Marcus, L.M., & Olley, J.G. (1980). The social and symbolic quality of autistic children's communication. *Journal of Autism and Developmental Disorders, 10*, 299–310.

Mesibov, G.B., Adams, L.W., & Klinger, L.G. (1997). *Autism: Understanding the disorder.* New York: Plenum Press.

Mesibov, G.B., Shea, V., & Adams, L.W. (2001). *Understanding Asperger syndrome and high-functioning autism.* New York: Kluwer Academic/Plenum Press.

Minshew, N.M., Goldstein, G., & Siegel, D.J. (1995). Speech and language in high-functioning autistic individuals. *Neuropsychology, 9*, 255–261.

Minshew, N.J., Goldstein, G., Taylor, G.H., & Siegel, D.J. (1994). Academic achievement in high functioning autistic individuals. *Journal of Clinical and Experimental Neuropsychology, 16*, 261–270.

Mirenda, P.L. (1997). Supporting individuals with challenging behavior through functional communication training and AAC: A research review. *AAC: Augmentative and Alternative Communication, 13*, 207–225.

Mirenda, P.L. (2001). Autism, augmentative communication, and assistive technology: What do we really know? *Focus on Autism and Other Developmental Disabilities, 16*, 141–151.

Mirenda, P.L. & Donnellan, A.M. (1986). Effects of adult interaction style on conversational behavior in students with severe communication problems. *Language, Speech, and Hearing Services in Schools, 17*, 126–141.

Mirenda, P.L. & Erickson, K.A. (2000). Augmentative communication and literacy. In A.M. Wetherby & B.M. Prizant (Eds.), *Autism spectrum disorders: A transactional developmental perspective* (pp. 333–367). Baltimore: Paul Brookes.

Nation, K. (1999). Reading skills in hyperlexia: A developmental perspective. *Psychological Bulletin, 125*, 338–355.

Peterson, S.L., Bondy, A.S., Vincent, Y., & Finnegan, C.S. (1995). Effects of altering communicative input for students with autism and no speech: Two case studies. *AAC: Augmentative and Alternative Communication, 11*, 93–100.

Pierce, S. & Bartolucci, G. (1977). A syntactic investigation of verbal autistic, mentally retarded, and normal children. *Journal of Autism and Developmental Disorders, 7*, 121–134.

Prizant, B.M. & Duchan, J.F. (1981). The functions of immediate echolalia in autistic children. *Journal of Speech and Hearing Disorders, 46*, 241–249.

Prizant, B.M. & Rydell, P.J. (1984). Analysis of functions of delayed echolalia in autistic children. *Journal of Speech and Hearing Research, 27*, 183–192.

Prizant, B.M., Schuler, A.L., Wetherby, A.M., & Rydell, P. (1997). Enhancing language and communication development: Language approaches. In D.J. Cohen & F.R. Volkmar (Eds.), *Handbook of autism and pervasive developmental disorders* (2nd ed.). (pp. 572–605). New York: John Wiley and Sons.

Prizant, B.M. & Wetherby, A.M. (1987). Communicative intent: A framework for understanding social-communicative behavior in autism. *Journal of the American Academy of Child and Adolescent Psychiatry, 26*, 472–479.

Prizant, B.M. & Wetherby, A.M. (1998). Understanding the continuum of discrete-trial traditional behavioral to social-pragmatic developmental approaches in communication enhancement for young children with autism/PDD. *Seminars in Speech & Language, 19*, 329–352.

Prizant, B.M., Wetherby, A.M., & Rydell, P.J. (2000). Communication intervention issues for young children with autism spectrum disorders. In A.M. Wetherby & B.M. Prizant (Eds.), *Autism spectrum disorders: A transactional developmental perspective* (pp. 193–224). Baltimore: Paul Brookes.

Rogers, S.J. (1996). Brief report: Early intervention in autism. *Journal of Autism and Developmental Disorders, 26*, 243–246.

Rollins, P.R., Wambacq, I., Dowell, D., Mathews, L., & Reese, P.B. (1998). An intervention technique for children with autistic spectrum disorder: Joint attentional routines. *Journal of Communication Disorders, 31*, 181–193.

Rydell, P.J. & Mirenda, P. (1994). Effects of high and low constraint utterances on the production of immediate and delayed echolalia in young children with autism. *Journal of Autism and Developmental Disorders, 24*, 719–735.

Sarokoff, R.A., Taylor, B.A., & Poulson, C.L. (2001). Teaching children with autism to engage in conversational exchanges: Script fading with embedded textual stimuli. *Journal of Applied Behavior Analysis, 34*, 81–84.

Schairer, K.S. & Nelson, N.W. (1996). Communicative possibilities of written conversations with adolescents who have autism. *Child Language Teaching and Therapy, 12*, 164–180

Schopler, E., Mesibov, G.B., & Kunce, L.J. (Eds.). (1998). *Asperger syndrome or high- functioning autism?* New York: Plenum Press.

Schuler, A.L. & Baldwin, M. (1981). Nonspeech communication and childhood autism. *Language, Speech, and Hearing Services in Schools, 12*, 246–257.

Schuler, A.L., Prizant, B.M., & Wetherby, A.M. (1997). Enhancing language and communication development: Prelinguistic approaches. In D.J. Cohen & F.R. Volkmar (Eds.), *Handbook of autism and pervasive developmental disorders* (2nd ed.). (pp. 539–571). New York: John Wiley and Sons.

Schwartz, I.S., Garfinkle, A.N., & Bauer, J. (1998). The picture exchange communication system: Communicative outcomes for young children with disabilities. *Topics in Early Childhood Special Education, 18*, 144–159.

Seal, B.C. & Bonvillian, J.D. (1997). Sign language and motor functioning in students with autistic disorder. *Journal of Autism and Developmental Disorders, 27*, 437–466.

Seibert, J.M. & Oller, D.K. (1981). Linguistic pragmatics and language intervention strategies. *Journal of Autism and Developmental Disorders, 11*, 75–88.

Shinner, S., Rapin, I., Arnold, S., Tuchman, R.F., Shulman, L., Ballaban-Gil, K. et al. (2001). Language regression in childhood. *Pediatric Neurology, 24*, 183–189.

Sigman, M. & Ruskin, E. (1999). Continuity and change in the social competence of children with autism, Down syndrome, and developmental delays. *Monographs of the Society for Research in Child Development* No 56, Vol 64.

Siller, M. & Sigman, M. (2002). The behaviors of parents of children with autism predict the subsequent development of their children's communication. *Journal of Autism and Developmental Disorders, 32*, 77–89.

Snyder-McLean, L.K., Solomonson, B., McLean, J.E., & Sack, S. (1984). Structuring joint action routines: A strategy for facilitating communication and language development in the classroom. *Seminars in Speech and Language, 5*, 213–228.

Stiebel, D. (1999). Promoting augmentative communication during daily routines. *Journal of Positive Behavior Interventions, 1*, 159–169.

Stone, W.L. & Caro-Martinez, L.M. (1990). Naturalistic observations of spontaneous communication in autistic children. *Journal of Autism and Developmental Disorders, 20*, 437–453.

Stone, W.L., Ousley, O.Y., Yoder, P.J., Hogan, K.L., & Hepburn, S.L. (1997). Nonverbal communication in two- and three-year old children with autism. *Journal of Autism and Developmental Disorders, 27*, 677–696.

Stone, W.L. & Yoder, P.J. (2001). Predicting spoken language level in children with autism spectrum disorders. *Autism, 5*, 341–361.

Swisher, L. & Demetras, M.J. (1985). The expressive language characteristics of autistic children compared with mentally retarded or specific language-impaired children. In E. Schopler & G.B. Mesibov (Eds.), *Communication Problems in Autism* (pp. 147–162). New York: Plenum Press.

Tager-Flusberg, H. (1981a). On the nature of linguistic functioning in early infantile autism. *Journal of Autism and Developmental Disorders, 11*, 45–56.

Tager-Flusberg, H. (1981b). Sentence comprehension in autistic children. *Applied Psycholinguistics, 2*, 5–24.

Tager-Flusberg, H. (1994). Dissociations in form and function in the acquisition of language by autistic children. In H. Tager-Flusberg (Ed.), *Constraints on language acquisition: Studies of atypical children.* (pp. 175–194). Hillsdale, NJ, US: Lawrence Erlbaum.

Tager-Flusberg, H. (1997). Perspectives on language and communication in autism. In D.J. Cohen & F.R. Volkmar (Eds.), *Handbook of autism and pervasive developmental disorders* (2nd ed.) (pp. 894–900). New York: John Wiley and Sons.

Tager-Flusberg, H. (2001). Understanding the language and communicative impairments in autism. *International Review of Research in Mental Retardation, 23*, 185–205.

Tager-Flusberg, H., Calkins, S., Nolin, T., Baumberger, T., Anderson, M., & Chadwick-Dias, A. (1990). A longitudinal study of language acquisition in autistic and Down syndrome children. *Journal of Autism and Developmental Disorders, 20*, 1–21.

Twachtman, D.D. (1995). Methods to enhance communication in verbal children. In K.A. Quill (Ed.), *Teaching children with autism: Strategies to enhance communication and socialization* (pp. 133–162). New York: Delmar.

Twachtman-Cullen, D.D. (2000). More able children with autism spectrum disorders: Sociocommunicative challenges and guidelines for enhancing abilities. In A.M. Wetherby & B.M. Prizant (Eds.), *Autism spectrum disorders: A transactional developmental perspective* (pp. 225–249). Baltimore: Paul Brookes.

Volden, J. & Lord, C. (1991). Neologisms and idiosyncratic language in autistic speakers. *Journal of Autism and Developmental Disorders, 21*, 109–130.

Watson, L.R. (1998). Following the child's lead: Mothers' interactions with children with autism. *Journal of Autism and Developmental Disorders, 28*, 51–59.

Watson, L.R., Lord, C., Schaffer, B. & Schopler, E. (1989). *Teaching spontaneous communication to autistic and developmentally handicapped children.* Austin, TX: Pro- Ed.

Wetherby, A.M. (1986). Ontogeny of communicative functions in autism. *Journal of Autism and Developmental Disorders, 16*, 295–316.

Wetherby, A.M., Prizant, B.M., & Schuler, A.L. (2000). Understanding the nature of communication and language impairments. In A.M. Wetherby & B.M. Prizant (Eds.), *Autism spectrum disorders: A transactional developmental perspective* (109–141). Baltimore: Paul Brookes.

Wetherby, A.M. & Prutting, C.A. (1984). Profiles of communicative and cognitive-social abilities in autistic children. *Journal of Speech and Hearing Research, 37*, 364–377.

Wetherby, A.M., Schuler, A.L., & Prizant, B.M. (1997). Enhancing language and communication development: Theoretical foundations. In D.J. Cohen & F.R. Volkmar (Eds.), *Handbook of autism and pervasive developmental disorders* (2nd ed.). (pp. 513–538). New York: John Wiley and Sons.

Wing, L. & Gould, J. (1979). Severe impairments of social interaction and associated abnormalities in children: Epidemiology and classification. *Journal of Autism and Developmental Disorders, 9*, 11–29.

Yoder, P.J. & Layton, T.L. (1988). Speech following sign language training in autistic children with minimal verbal language. *Journal of Autism and Developmental Disorders, 18*, 217–229.

CHAPTER 7

Social Skills

INTRODUCTION

The social problems associated with autism spectrum disorders (ASD) are among the most complex and pervasive characteristics of this condition, because difficulties with interpersonal relationships involve problems in language, nonverbal communication, thinking, and understanding (Schopler & Mesibov, 1986). Difficulties interacting with others are seen in individuals with ASD of all ages and cognitive/developmental levels. Further, social problems occur in a variety of settings, including school or work, the community, and home. Improving social skills can enhance the ability of people with ASD to function successfully in their communities, and can also play an important role in enriching their personal lives.

In this chapter we will briefly review typical social development and examine the social characteristics of ASD. A representative sample of the literature on improving social skills in people with ASD will be covered (see McConnell, 2002 and Rogers, 2000 for more extensive reviews), and then the TEACCH approach to social skills will be discussed.

TYPCIAL DEVELOPMENT OF SOCIAL BEHAVIORS

For normally developing children, positive interpersonal experiences seem to be predetermined. Without deliberate training or planned exposure on the part of their parents, normal infants develop eye contact, respond to cuddling, are fascinated by human faces, and orient to human voices. Normally developing children also learn very early that others can satisfy an enormous number of their needs. Given this background, it is not surprising that normally developing children are extremely motivated to expand their social interactions. As typical development unfolds, children learn to interact with their parents in more complex ways, such as the social routines of 'peek-a-boo' and 'so big' and repeating behaviors that make their parents laugh. Young children also become interested in watching other children, imitating their behaviors, playing near them, doing what they do (that is, parallel play), and eventually learning to share materials, take turns, and play cooperatively and imaginatively. Later in development, social interactions typically become much more verbal, in the form of conversations about personal feelings and topics of mutual interest.

EFFECTS OF AUTISM SPECTRUM
DISORDERS ON SOCIAL BEHAVIORS

This sequence of social skill development does not occur in the same way or at the same time for children with ASD. Diagnostic criteria for both autism and Asperger Syndrome include impairments in behaviors such as eye-to-eye gaze, facial expression, body postures, gestures related to social interaction, and a lack of spontaneous seeking to share enjoyment, interest, or achievements with others (DSM-IV-TR; APA, 2000). Recent research has also shown that children with ASD in the first year of life can be distinguished by limited social responsiveness (Baranek, 1999; Maestro et al., 2002; Werner, Dawson, & Osterling, 2000).

So from an early age, children with ASD do not establish the typical foundations of understanding, trusting, and enjoying social interactions. This picture can deteriorate even further as youngsters with ASD grow older, because their lack of skills makes social situations frustrating or unpleasant. This situation must be reversed if individuals with ASD are ever to enjoy and appreciate social interactions.

Patterns of Observable Social Behavior in
Autism Spectrum Disorders

Wing and Gould (1979) described three different patterns of social behavior seen in individuals with ASD, and used the terms 'aloof,' 'passive,' and socially 'active but odd' to describe these patterns. The 'aloof' pattern refers to withdrawing from or actively rejecting social bids from others. The 'passive' pattern describes the behavior of individuals who generally accept social bids from others, but rarely initiate social contact, while the active but odd descriptor is used for individuals who actively seek out social interactions, but do so in unusual or very awkward ways. Later research has validated these constructs and has found that the 'aloof' pattern tends to be associated with mental retardation, while individuals with higher IQs are more likely to demonstrate the 'active but odd' pattern (Borden & Ollendick, 1994; O'Brien, 1996; Volkmar, Cohen, Bregman, Hooks, & Stevenson, 1989; Waterhouse et al., 1996). Wing (2000) has also described a fourth pattern of social interaction skills seen in some individuals with above-average intelligence, who display social skills based on rote learning.

Underlying Neuropsychological Patterns

Several neuropsychological characteristics of autism interfere with the ability to interact socially. First, as noted above, studies of early symptoms of autism identify pervasive deficits in these children's social skills, such as their ability to make eye contact with their primary caregivers (Swettenham et al., 1998) or orient to social stimuli (Dawson, Meltzoff, Osterling, Rinaldi, & Brown, 1998)

Second, for most individuals with ASD, motivation to initiate activity is low for social interactions, compared to initiation of non-social activities (Swettenham et al., 1998). This limited motivation adds to the challenge when offering social skills training for individuals with ASD (Klinger & Dawson, 1992; Pierce & Schreibman, 1995). However, it should again be noted that not all individuals with ASD are uninterested in social interactions; some still very much want to be a part of the social circles in their schools and communities. Unfortunately, however, lack of skills or inappropriate behavior often lead to social failures. These failures may be particularly difficult for older or more cognitively advanced individuals with ASD, who appear to be aware of their deficits in social functioning and unhappy about how those deficits isolate them (Capps, Sigman, & Yirmiya, 1995).

A third characteristic of ASD that has a negative impact on social relations is that when children with ASD *do* initiate interactions, these are likely to be routinized, rather than imitative or reciprocally interactive (Hauck, Fein, Waterhouse, & Feinstein, 1995). Such stilted and awkward initiations by children with autism can limit their ability to play with peers and make these interactions less satisfying or effective.

Fourth, children with ASD are not attuned to the subtleties of social rules and behaviors (Gray, 1998). For example, individuals with ASD have difficulty reading vocal and facial expressions, which might distinguish a serious statement from a sarcastic comment. People with ASD also have difficulty interpreting subtle gestural cues and reading body language, which might lead them to violate their peers' personal space and other boundaries.

Fifth, individuals with ASD also generally have difficulty understanding other people's perspectives, sometimes described as Theory of Mind deficits, and therefore are often unable to decipher what other people are thinking and the implications of these thoughts (Baron-Cohen, 2001). This deficit makes it difficult for them to understand and utilize social feedback. For example, a person with ASD may talk perseveratively about a special interest like cash registers, without considering or realizing that the peer is uninterested in or uninformed about the topic. Not looking for outward signals of others' reactions and not recognizing nonverbal cues, such as eye rolling, gaze shifting, or fidgeting, which indicate that the partner is getting bored, might contribute to the Theory of Mind problem. Further, difficulties with joint attention behaviors, such as making eye contact or following gaze or physical gestures, may compound Theory of Mind deficits (Mundy & Sigman, 1989; Rogers, 1998) by limiting the information available to the individual with ASD about the other person's state of mind or interests.

As a result of deficits in these 'prewired' social skills from an early age, an accelerating vicious cycle can develop. Limited knowledge, experience, motivation and skills can lead to being ignored or ostracized by peers, which then reduces opportunities to develop social skills. Research has suggested that such a lack of social experiences and skills may have a profound effect on the social adjustment of children (Hartup & Sancilio, 1986) and also hinder the long-term development of social communicative behavior (McGee, Morrier, & Daly, 1999).

INTERVENTION TECHNIQUES

A common foundation for social skills training for children and adults with disabilities is the concept of 'normalization' (Wolfensberger, 1972) which emphasizes the importance of teaching specific social skills so that the individuals with disabilities do not stand out, and are therefore more acceptable to their peers. Skills typically taught include behaviors such as making eye contact, asking or offering to share a toy, joining a group, giving compliments, etc. This approach is generally carried out using behavioral techniques, either in individual instruction or in groups.

Individual Instruction

A typical individual intervention technique involves teacher instruction using principles of behavior modification (Strain & Schwartz, 2001). Teachers use direct one-to-one training techniques (e.g., cueing, prompting, modeling, reinforcement) for developing specific social behaviors. Ideally, prompts are eventually faded out as students learn targeted skills. Then, in social settings, students are positively reinforced with consequences, such as attention, praise, or preferred items for engaging in specific appropriate social behaviors. In addition, teachers may arrange their classrooms in ways that make social activities motivating, which encourages children to initiate social behaviors (McGee, Morrier, & Daly, 1999). Studies have indicated that using teacher-mediated or one-to-one teaching techniques to initiate social interactions prior to practicing them with peers increases the frequency and duration of interactions (Gaylord-Ross & Haring, 1987; Gaylord-Ross, Haring, Breen, & Pitts-Conway, 1984).

Hwang and Hughes (2000) reviewed several behavioral strategies used with individual children to increase their social interactive skills. The strategies were contingent imitation, naturally occurring reinforcement, time delays, and environmental engagement. The authors reported that the four techniques were each effective, under certain circumstances, at teaching children a variety of skills. In addition, combining strategies and using different techniques for different skills increased treatment effectiveness. It seems that individualizing treatment, according to both the person and the skill being taught, is a way to increase the success of behavioral interventions.

However, because of the significant difficulty people with ASD have in generalizing learned skills from one situation to another, social skills must be practiced in naturalistic settings; it is difficult to simulate the range of real life social situations in a one-to-one format with a familiar teacher. For this reason, peer group intervention efforts have become more popular and are more widely implemented.

Group Interventions

The first group social skills intervention program for individuals with ASD reported in the literature was conducted by Mesibov (1984). This program promoted positive peer experiences as a way to increase interpersonal skills and improve self-concepts among adolescents and adults with relatively good cognitive skills (IQs above 60). The groups met weekly for $1\frac{1}{2}$ hours each week over a 24-week period. Group sessions were preceded by individual one-on-one practice sessions emphasizing the skills to be practiced that week. Interventions followed a cognitive behavioral model, including discussions and explanations of the skills studied and the reasons for them, modeling, coaching, and role-playing. The author reports that based on family and participant judgments of change, the program was successful.

Williams (1989) described a similar social skills program several years later. This was a long-term group, including 10 participants over a period of several years. The group focused on perspective taking, conversational skills, and flexibility. Brainstorming, modeling, games, and role-play were the main intervention strategies. Williams reported that limited progress occurred in perspective taking and some of the other specific skills, but more general measures of social skills and behaviors showed improvement. The main areas that showed progress were talking with peers, initiating conversations with staff, and related social and conversational skills.

Several other group intervention programs have also been reported in the literature. Working with younger (age 8–12) children with Asperger syndrome, Marriage, Gordon, and Brand (1995) found increases in self-confidence and the acquisition of some concrete social skills, but no generalization to other settings. Howlin and Yates (1999) reported improvements in adults as a result of their social groups and Ozonoff and Miller (1995) were able to elicit changes in perspective-taking ability of adolescents autism and average intelligence, although these individuals had difficulty with generalization outside the treatment settings as well.

Organizing principles for conducting social groups are clearly articulated by Krasny, Williams, Provencal, and Ozonoff (2003). These include making the abstract concrete, providing structure and predictability, providing scaffolded language support, providing multiple and varied learning opportunities, including "other"-focused activities, fostering self-awareness and self-esteem, selecting relevant goals, programming in a sequential and progressive manner, and providing opportunities for programmed generalization and on-going practice.

Limitations of Skill Training

Although children with ASD can improve their social functioning following skill-based training programs emphasizing normalized behaviors, children in these programs still demonstrate lower levels of motivation to engage in social interactions than their typically developing peers, have a more limited understanding of social expectations, and have less social experience. Therefore, the skills that they learn often do not generalize to other settings and may eventually fade away (Schopler & Mesibov, 1986).

In addition, several reports suggest that isolated and specific social skills do not account for the social interaction problems so commonly observed in youngsters with ASD. Atwood, Frith and Hermelin (1988) found no differences between children with ASD and a control group with Down syndrome in the use of instrumental gestures, when the amount of time spent interacting was controlled. Magill and Lord (1989) reported that specific social behaviors such as eye contact were as frequent in high-functioning people with ASD as in non-handicapped controls. Both studies, however, found major differences in the frequency of social interactions. Thus, the presence of specific social behaviors does not necessarily predict actual social success.

Further, research has not demonstrated a clear relationship between acquisition of social skills and acceptance by peers of children with disabilities (Hurley-Geffner, 1995), suggesting that despite possible improvement in overall social skills, children with ASD are not necessarily better liked or more accepted by their peers.

In summary, the literature indicates that there is some, but limited value, in teaching isolated components of social behavior, particularly in learning situations which then must be generalized to other settings in order to be used.

THE TEACCH APPROACH

Goals

The TEACCH approach to social skills training, like other aspects of TEACCH's work, has the ultimate goal of helping people with ASD to function as well and as independently as possible given their individual circumstances. Accomplishing this goal rests on a foundation of the empirical research literature, an understanding of the characteristics of autism (see Chapter 3, The

Culture of Autism), and consideration of the individual's strengths, needs, and personal interests.

Unlike programs that focus on teaching individual social behaviors, however, the priority for TEACCH's work in the area of social skills is making play and socializing enjoyable. Positive experiences with other people are an important foundation for the development of social skills in individuals who have limited interest, understanding, and experience in social interactions. Thus, the fundamental goal is creating and repeatedly practicing personally meaningful experiences in social contexts, rather than teaching specific social behaviors that might make an individual appear more 'normal' (Garfin & Lord, 1986). If this important goal is accomplished, then specific behaviors such as eye contact and smiling may follow, if they are truly essential for meaningful interactions (Lord & Magill, 1989).

Even for individuals who are interested in social participation but whose attempts are often met with rejection, it is important that the social group experiences be interesting, exciting, and informative. Although for these participants the issue is not one of limited motivation to interact socially, it is important for their feelings of well-being and self-confidence that they be accepted by a group of peers whom they perceive as desirable and interesting.

Techniques

Individual Interests

The most important technique for making social interactions enjoyable is using the interests and understanding of the participants to guide activities. Because individuals with ASD often reject social opportunities from lack of interest, making social activities enjoyable is crucial for increasing motivation to engage in these activities. This is true regardless of the individual's age or functioning level. For example, when working with young children with ASD, we do not emphasize specific skills such as looking at the other child simply because normal children engage in that behavior. Although the research literature indicates that this skill can be taught, it also suggests that the skill of making eye contact does not necessarily predict increased social aptitude. In our view, it is more important to keep the children working or playing near or with other children on activities at all levels that are interesting and meaningful to them.

Activities that we have found to be enjoyable for various individuals are listed below:

Young children and concrete learners
Simple play with their favorite materials (either parallel play or very easy activities such as handing materials to each other, taking turns tossing materials into a basket, taking turns placing puzzle pieces, etc.), follow the leader, rolling a ball or truck back and forth, sharing snacks, singing songs

School-aged children and concrete learners
   Musical chairs, simple board games, crafts or art activities, playing to-
   gether with sand or in water
Teens and young adults
   Bingo, watching movies, videogames, conversations, eating out together,
   bowling
Adults
   Going to movies, sporting activities, restaurants, playing social games
   such as Scrabble or cards, discussing social issues, attending concerts

Highly Structured Groups

Much of the work on social behavior is done in the setting in which skills
eventually are to be used; that is, in social groups. Groups vary in size, however,
depending on the personalities, skills, and needs of participants. For example,
for younger and/or people with more severe cognitive or interpersonal disabilities, a group can have as few as two people. Older and more capable individuals
can often participate in and benefit from groups as large as 10–15 peers.

Groups typically involve a combination of shared recreational activities
such as those listed above, and for older and more capable learners, structured
interactions (such as practicing solutions to conflicts at work, or asking a potential friend to have coffee) and occasional free conversation. Within all groups,
practice and multiple opportunities to interact are essential.

To be effective, groups must be highly structured and individualized. Principles and techniques of Structured Teaching are used with each participant
with ASD (see Chapter 4, Structured Teaching). Each participant is given the
visual structure he or she needs for learning and using social skills (such as
charts, checklists, or conversational pointers or scripts). Thus, for example,
instead of verbally or physically prompting the student with ASD to play a
game, we would prepare visual directions in advance, and use visual prompts
as needed. For instance, a teacher may place a set of playing cards in a folder with
directions for the game "Go Fish" written out, along with an object to be passed
back and forth to indicate whose turn it was. Although a typically-developing
person may understand the game based on a verbal explanation alone, the individual with ASD is likely to comprehend the directions and the sequence of
the game better when this information is provided visually.

Some of our youngest or most aloof, socially handicapped individuals have
very basic social experiences in these groups, such as learning to play with
familiar materials in the same physical location as another person. No demands
for social interactions are made, and the individual is provided with visual
information that indicates *where* to be (for example, the person is seated in a
chair or the play area is clearly marked on the floor with colored tape), *what* to
do (a familiar toy or favorite materials are in a basket), *how long* to do it (a timer
is set; the ticking shows progress toward the end, and when it rings, the play
session is finished), and what will happen *next* (there is a different basket to
put the play materials in, and a cup to direct the person to the snack table).

As the social comfort and skills of these children improve, goals can be increased. For example, two individuals who have learned an activity with a teacher (such as handing puzzle pieces to each other, or alternating turning over cards) would be asked to do the activity with each other, again with the visual structure to show them 'where, what, how long, how to know they are making progress toward a clear finish, and what to do next.' The next step for one individual might be to find a partner with whom to do the same activity, in a situation where partners are obviously available. The next step for a different individual might be learning to play different games with the same partner. A third individual might learn to respond to conversational bids while playing the game. Eventually the goal might be to enter a room and find someone to play with or talk with. This process mirrors the approach of skill-based training that fades teacher or peer prompts to enable the person with ASD to become more independent in interactions. The key differences in the TEACCH approach are 1) selecting activities that are highly motivating to the individual learners; 2) using visual structure so that the activities are visually clear and meaningful; and 3) increasing positive social experiences in meaningful contexts.

Typically-developing Peers

We have often found that typically-developing peers can positively influence the learning of people with ASD, so we include them in our groups whenever possible. However, simply placing typical peers and individuals with ASD together is not sufficient; several important steps are necessary to make this integrated experience of maximum benefit (Mesibov, 1976; McHale & Gamble, 1986).

When working with youngsters, it is extremely important that the neurotypical peers be well-prepared before the social interactions. Preparation includes a general explanation of autism along with specific suggestions of activities that are appropriate for the children with ASD they will be directly working with. Suggestions about particular materials and activities, such as 'Johnny enjoys catching a nerf ball' or 'Bob likes to draw cartoon characters' are the most effective. The focus is on providing enjoyable, meaningful experiences for the individuals with ASD, so that the activities make sense to them, while making these activities enjoyable and roles clear for the nonhandicapped participants as well.

One difficulty revealed by research into peer-mediated interventions is keeping the neurotypical children motivated to continue initiating interactions with the peer with ASD (Schopler & Mesibov, 1986). Part of this problem stems from the peers' difficulty understanding the unusual behaviors of the children with ASD. We have several ways of helping the non-handicapped peers. A general suggestion we make is that if they can't figure out what the child with ASD is doing, they should imitate the activity and then gradually make it a little more interesting when the youngster with ASD is watching them. For example, if the child with ASD runs around the play area, first follow him and then begin to change the route gradually in ways that make it fun and interesting. We also suggest that peers working with children try to stay on the same physical level, such as standing up or lying down when the child with ASD does this, so that the opportunity for social interaction is maintained. We suggest that peers should show the children with ASD what they want and how to do things, rather than just making verbal suggestions. Also, imitating a child with ASD can be an effective strategy for attracting his or her attention. Finally, we emphasize the need for persistence: sometimes the typically-developing peers will have to try several times to get their playmates' attention or cooperation.

In addition, peers may have some difficulty comprehending the goals of their interactions or how to make the activities enjoyable. Regular opportunities for the peers to discuss their ideas, questions, and concerns with group leaders are provided. This is especially important if some of the participants with ASD exhibit unusual behaviors or tantrums.

Conversational Guidelines

Although many older or more verbal individuals with ASD have favorite topics and are able to communicate about them, they often have difficulty building their interests into acceptable interpersonal opportunities. They may talk about their interests to excess, and lose the attention of their conversational partner. For example, idiosyncratic interests such as shoes, people's birthdays, transportation schedules, and specific sporting events might be appropriate topics for brief conversation for neurotypical adults, but they are rarely pursued for the length of time and with the degree of detail that characterizes the conversation of individuals with ASD. An effective approach to teaching conversational skills to such individuals is to use their interests to motivate conversations and interactions, but then help the participants understand how much is too much (Mesibov, 1984). In social groups organized by TEACCH, we often pair participants with non-handicapped peers of approximately the same age to discuss topics that each participant is interested in. Later, we teach conversational guidelines such as "after 3 sentences about the topic you like to learn about, ask your partner what he/she likes to learn about." Another technique is to change topics every 3 minutes, rotating who selects the topic. We might also generate a list of 10 topics that are typically discussed by individuals of a particular age and have the participants pick a topic from that list for them to talk about. (See also Chapter 6, Communication).

Teacher or Staff Involvement

We have found it helpful for staff to be directly involved with the group activities as participants. This adds to the enjoyment, especially for groups of older children and adults. It also enables the staff to directly model appropriate activities and specific social strategies to support the neurotypical peers when things are difficult. A positive and enthusiastic approach to these sessions is essential for all staff members.

In making this a positive experience for the typical peers, it is important not to overestimate their involvement or level of interaction. Although peers often find these groups to be extremely positive and meaningful, it is important to remember that these groups are not the same experience for them as playing with their friends. Assuming that the relationships in these groups will provide the same intrinsic satisfaction as self-selected friendships could lead to underestimating the need for careful preparation described above and the support and external reinforcement that are necessary to maintain these groups.

Therefore, the leaders' roles in these activities is both maintaining the positive tone of the activities for handicapped and non-handicapped peers, as well as helping to provide structure for some activities that may be difficult for individuals with autism to understand.

CONCLUDING COMMENTS

The primary goal of TEACCH social interventions is to make social interactions interesting, meaningful, and positive for individuals with ASD. Therefore, rather than targeting specific skills to make the participants appear 'normal,' we target understanding and enjoyment of activities in social settings, and thus increase the likelihood that social settings and social interactions will become pleasant and desirable. These strategies also increase the amount of practice students with ASD get in social interactions. Our experiences have demonstrated that this approach can help individuals of all ages and skills levels with ASD to enjoy social situations and improve their social skills in the process.

REFERENCES

American Psychiatric Association. (2000). *Diagnostic and statistical manual of mental disorders (4th ed., Text Revision)*. Washington, DC: Author.

Attwood, T., Frith, U., & Hermelin, B. (1988). The understanding and use of interpersonal gestures by autistic and Down's syndrome children. *Journal of Autism and Developmental Disorders, 18*, 241–257.

Baranek, G. (1999). Autism during infancy: A retrospective video analysis of sensory-motor and social behaviors at 9–12 months of age. *Journal of Autism and Developmental Disorders, 29*, 213–224.

Baron-Cohen, S. (2001). Theory of mind and autism: A review. In L.M. Glidden (Ed). *International review of research in mental retardation: Autism (vol. 23)* (pp. 169–184). San Diego, CA: Academic Press.

Borden, M.C. & Ollendick, T.H. (1994). An examination of the validity of social subtypes in autism. *Journal of Autism and Developmental Disorders, 24*, 23–27.

Capps, L., Sigman, M., & Yirmiya, N. (1995). Self-competence and emotional understanding in high-functioning children with autism. *Development and Psychopathology, 7*, 137–149.

Dawson, G., Meltzoff, A.N., Osterling, J., Rinaldi, J., & Brown, E. (1998). Children with autism fail to orient to naturally occurring social stimuli. *Journal of Autism and Developmental Disorders, 28*, 479–485.

Garfin, D. & Lord, C. (1986). Communication as a social problem in autism. In E. Schopler & G.B. Mesibov (Eds.), *Social behavior in autism* (pp. 237–261). New York: Plenum Press.

Gaylord-Ross, R. & Haring, T. (1987). Social interaction research for adolescents with severe handicaps. *Behavioral Disorders, 12*, 264–275

Gaylord-Ross, R., Haring, T.G., Breen, C., & Pitts-Conway, V. (l984). The training and generalization of social interaction skills with autistic youth. *Journal of Applied Behavior Analysis, 17,* 229–247.

Gray, C.A. (1998). Social stories and comic strip conversations with students with Asperger syndrome and high-functioning autism. In E. Schopler, G.B. Mesibov, & L.J. Kunce (Eds.), *Asperger syndrome or high-functioning autism?* (pp. 167–198). New York: Plenum Press.

Hartup, W.W. & Sancilio, M.F. (1986). Children's friendships. In E. Schopler & G.B. Mesibov (Eds.), *Social behavior in autism* (pp. 61–79). New York: Plenum Press.

Hauck, M., Fein, D., Waterhouse, L., & Feinstein, C. (1995). Social initiations by autistic children to adults and other children. *Journal of Autism and Developmental Disorders, 25,* 579–595.

Howlin P. & Yates, P. (1999). The potential effectiveness of social skills groups for adults with autism. *Autism, 3,* 299–307.

Hurley-Geffner, C.M. (1995). Friendships between children with and without developmental disabilities. In R.L. Koegel & L.K. Koegel (Eds.), *Teaching children with autism: Strategies for initiating positive interactions and improving learning opportunities* (pp. 105–125). Baltimore: Paul H. Brookes.

Hwang, B. & Hughes, C. (2000). The effects of social interaction training on early social communicative skills of children with autism. *Journal of Autism and Developmental Disorders, 30,* 331–343.

Klinger, L.G. & Dawson, G. (1992). Facilitating early social and communicative development in children with autism. In S.F. Warren & J.E. Reichle (Eds.), *Causes and effects in communication and language intervention* (pp. 157–186). Baltimore: Paul H. Brookes.

Krasny, L., Williams, B., Provencal, S., & Ozonoff, S. (2003). Social skills interventions for the autism spectrum: Essential ingredients and a model curriculum. *Child and Adolescent Psychiatric Clinics of North America, 12,* 107–122.

Lord, C. & Hopkins, J.M. (1986). The social behavior of autistic children with younger and same-age nonhandicapped peers. *Journal of Autism & Developmental Disorders, 16,* 249–262

Lord, C. & Magill, J. (1989). Methodological and theoretical issues in studying peer-directed behavior and autism. In G. Dawson (Ed.), *Autism: New perspectives on diagnosis, nature, and treatment* (pp. 326–345). New York: Guilford Press.

Maestro, S., Muratori, F., Cavallaro, M.C., Pei, F., Stern, D., Golse, B. et al. (2002). Attentional skills during the first 6 months of age in autism spectrum disorder. *Journal of the American Academy of Child & Adolescent Psychiatry, 41,* 1239–1245.

Magill, J. & Lord, C. (1987). An observational study of greetings of autistic, behavior-disordered, and normally-developing children (unpublished manuscript).

Marriage, K.J., Gordon, V., & Brand, L. (1995). A social skills group for boys with Asperger's syndrome. *Australian and New Zealand Journal of Psychiatry, 29,* 58–62.

McConnell, S.R. (2002). Interventions to facilitate social interaction for young children with autism: Review of available research and recommendations for educational intervention and future research. *Journal of Autism and Developmental Disorders, 32,* 351–372.

McGee, G.G., Morrier, M., & Daly, T. (1999). An incidental teaching approach to early intervention for toddlers with autism. *Journal of the Association for Persons with Severe Handicaps, 24,* 133–146.

McHale, S.M. & Gamble, W.C. (1986). Mainstreaming handicapped children in public school settings: Challenges and limitations. In E. Schopler & G.B. Mesibov (Eds.), *Social behavior in autism* (pp. 191–212). New York: Plenum Press.

Mesibov, G.B (1976). Implications of the normalization principle for psychotic children. *Journal of Autism & Childhood Schizophrenia, 6,* 360–364.

Mesibov, G.B. (1984). Social skills training with verbal autistic adolescents and adults: A program model. *Journal of Autism and Developmental Disorders, 14,* 395–404.

Myles, B.S., Simpson, R.L., Ormsbee, C.K., & Erickson, C. (1993). Integrating preschool children with autism with their normally developing peers: Research findings and best practices recommendations. *Focus on Autistic Behavior, 8,* 1–18.

Mundy, P. & Sigman, M. (1989). The theoretical implications of joint attention deficits in autism. *Development and Psychopathology, 1,* 173–183.

O'Brien, S.K. (1996). The validity and reliability of the Wing Subgroups Questionnaire. *Journal of Autism and Developmental Disabilities, 26*, 321–335.

Ozonoff, S. & Miller, J. (1995). Teaching theory of mind: A new approach to social skills training for individuals with autism. *Journal of Autism and Developmental Disorders, 25*, 415–433.

Pierce, K. & Schreibman, L. (1995). Increasing complex social behaviors in children with autism: Effects of peer-implemented pivotal response training. *Journal of Applied Behavior Analysis, 28*, 285–295.

Rogers, S.J. (1998). Neuropsychology of autism in young children and its implications for early intervention. *Mental Retardation and Developmental Disabilities Research Reviews, 4*, 104–112.

Rogers, S.J. (2000). Interventions that facilitate socialization in children with autism. *Journal of Autism and Developmental Disorders, 30*, 399–409.

Schopler, E. & Mesibov, G.B. (Eds.). (1986). *Social behavior in autism.* New York: Plenum Press.

Strain, P.S. & Schwartz, I. (2001). ABA and the development of meaningful social relations for young children with autism. *Focus on Autism and Other Developmental Disabilities, 16*, 120–128.

Swettenham, J., Baron-Cohen, S., Charman, T., Cox, A., Baird, G., Drew, A., et al. (1998). The frequency and distribution of spontaneous attention shifts between social and nonsocial stimuli in autistic, typically developing, and nonautistic developmentally delayed infants. *Journal of Child Psychology and Psychiatry and Allied Disciplines, 39*, 747–753.

Volkmar, F.R., Cohen, D.J., Bregman, J.D., Hooks, M.Y., & Stevenson, J.M. (1989). An examination of social typologies found in autism. *Journal of the American Academy of Child and Adolescent Psychiatry, 28*, 82–86.

Waterhouse, L., Morris, R., Allen, D., Dunn, M., Fein, D., Feinstein, C., et al. (1996). Diagnosis and classification in autism. *Journal of Autism and Developmental Disorders, 26*, 59–86.

Werner, E., Dawson, G., Osterling, J., & Dinno, N. (2000). Brief report: Recognition of autism spectrum disorder before one year of age: A retrospective study based on home videotapes. *Journal of Autism and Developmental Disorders, 30*, 157–162.

Williams, T.I. (1989). A social skills group for autistic children. *Journal of Autism and Developmental Disorders, 19*, 143–155.

Wing, L. (2000). Past and future of research on autism. In. A. Klin, F.R.Volkmar, & S.S. Sparrow (Eds.). *Asperger syndrome* (pp. 418–432). New York: Guilford Press.

Wing L. & Gould, J. (1979). Severe impairments of social interaction and associated abnormalities in children: Epidemiology and classification. *Journal of Autism and Developmental Disorders, 9*, 11–29.

Wolfensberger, W. (1972). *The principle of normalization in human services.* Toronto, Ontario, Canada: National Institute on Mental Retardation.

CHAPTER 8

Parents

HISTORICAL BACKGROUND

In the paper in which Leo Kanner (1943) first described the 11 young patients he labeled autistic, he also discussed his observations about their parents. Kanner indicated that all of the parents were highly intelligent and well-educated. He also described these parents as sharing a number of personality characteristics, which he depicted in fairly negative terms.

Over the years, Kanner struggled with the speculation that parents' personalities and interactions with their children caused autism. On the one hand, in his original paper he wrote that "the children's aloneness from the beginning of life makes it difficult to attribute the whole picture exclusively to the type of the early parental relations with our patients. We must, then, assume that these children have come into the world with innate inability to form the usual, biologically provided affective contact with people, just as other children come into the world with innate physical or intellectual handicaps" (1943, p. 250). On the other hand, after describing his negative view of the parents' personalities and marriages in this same paper, he stated that "the question arises whether or to what extent this . . . has contributed to the condition of the children" (1943, p. 250). He wrote other articles (Eisenberg and Kanner, 1956; Kanner, 1949) that also indicated that parents were responsible for autism. However, in later years Kanner (1968) modified this view, focusing again on the inborn, biological nature of autism.

While Kanner vacillated about the role of parents in their child's autism, the major factor in the development of the inaccurate and unproductive view of parents' responsibility for autism was the work of Bruno Bettelheim (1967). Although Bettelheim was widely assumed to be a psychiatrist, in fact he was neither a physician, nor a psychologist, nor a trained psychoanalyst (Pollack, 1997). He studied art history and international commerce, earned a degree in aesthetics from the University of Vienna, and was working in his father's lumber business in Vienna when World War II began. After 11 months in a concentration camp, in 1939 he was allowed to emigrate to the United States, where he presented himself as a child therapist and soon rose to prominence in the field of child psychopathology, eventually becoming the Director of the Orthogenic School at the University of Chicago. As described in Chapter 1 (The Origins and History of the TEACCH Program), Bettelheim had extremely negative views of the parents of children with autism. His policy was to separate those children from their parents and exclude the parents from the children's treatment, which resulted in monumental parental guilt and ineffective 'therapy' for both parents and children. However, his prolific writing, media appearances, and exaggerated claims made him a very influential figure for many decades, both in the professional training of child psychologists and psychiatrists, educators, and other professionals, and also in the popular culture, which further spread the erroneous notion that parental pathology caused autism.

CHANGING PERSPECTIVES

By the mid-late 1960's, some professionals were beginning to question the prevailing theory that parents caused autism, and research began to accumulate that autism is a biologically-based disorder (Ornitz & Ritvo, 1968; Rimland, 1964; Rutter, 1965, 1968; Schopler, 1966; Wing, 1966). Among the earliest professionals to disagree with the view that autism was a reaction to pathological parenting were the co-founders of the TEACCH program, psychologist Eric Schopler and psychiatrist Robert Reichler (See Chapter 1, The Origins and History of the TEACCH Program). Schopler and Reichler based their work on the assumption that parents of youngsters with autism were typical people struggling valiantly with the challenges and burdens of raising their developmentally disabled children without much professional support or assistance (Schopler, 1997).

In 1965 a national parents' group, the National Society for Autistic Children, was formed (it is now the Autism Society of America), to provide support and information-exchange among parents and professionals and to advocate for the needs of individuals with autism (Warren, 1984). The attitude of most professionals toward parents became more supportive and respectful, and beginning in the mid-1970's a number of researchers began to examine patterns of stress and coping among parents of children with autism.

Studies of Stress and Coping

Conclusive results from the body of research into parents' stress and coping strategies have been limited by various methodological factors, such as small samples, wide age ranges of the 'children,' samples that may not be representative of the population of parents or of children with carefully diagnosed ASD, and a large number of measurement instruments that may not be comparable to each other. Still, some general trends have emerged from the research literature.

Interviews

Several studies based on interviews with autism parents from different areas of the world revealed similar concerns and experiences. Using a semi-structured interview technique, Midence and O'Neill (1999) talked with parents of children with autism in Wales about their experiences and identified in their responses six shared themes: 1) the unusual behavior and development of their children; 2) the strain of not understanding their children or knowing what was wrong with them, which led to feelings of worry and guilt; 3) difficulty obtaining a correct diagnosis; 4) relief and increased clarity when a diagnosis was made; 5) the importance of help and support from experts; and 6) the eventual adaptation of the family to enjoyment and appreciation of their children.

Interviews with parents of adolescents with autism in Alberta, Canada (Fong, Wilgosh, & Sobsey, 1993) yielded six areas of common concern: 1) difficult behaviors, including "temper tantrums and aggressive, self-abusive, destructive, obsessive, ritualistic, impulsive, and self-stimulatory behaviors" (p. 108); 2) limited social skills and judgment that often resulted in being teased or rejected; 3) the effect of the youngster with autism on the family, such as financial strains and the need to provided "constant supervision and assistance with daily living skills" (p. 109); 4) the problems associated with school and related services; 5) stressful experiences with professionals; and 6) worries about the future, including living arrangements and sexuality. These families reported benefiting greatly from the support of their spouses, other families and friends, and their employers.

Kohler (1999) interviewed families of children with autism in a region of Pennsylvania, who reported concerns about delayed diagnosis, ineffective services and unmet needs, and poor communication and coordination among service providers. However, some parents also reported receiving exceptionally valuable services and information.

Rating Scales

Most studies using rating scales have found that autism parents, particularly mothers, report experiencing more stress than parents of typically developing children or those with Down Syndrome or other clinical conditions (Bebko, Konstantareas, & Springer, 1987; Bouma & Schweitzer, 1990; Dumas, Wolf, Fisman, & Culligan, 1991; Holroyd & McArthur, 1976; Hoppes & Harris, 1990; Koegel et al., 1992; Konstantareas, Homatidis, & Plowright, 1992; Rodrigue, Morgan, & Geffken, 1990, 1992; Sanders & Morgan, 1997; Sharpley, Bitsika, & Efremdis, 1997; Sivberg, 2002; Weiss, 2002). DeMyer and Goldberg (1983) reported that the most common concerns or negative effects of having a child with autism were in the family's ability to participate in recreational activities and in the areas of finances and the psychological well-being of the parents. Similarly, Fisman, Wolf, and Noh (1989) found that autism mothers in their sample rated their families significantly lower than mothers in the control groups on the items reflecting 'working and playing together comfortably.' Bristol (1987) also reported significantly more disruption of daily activities within families of children with autism or other developmental disabilities compared to typical families, a finding consistent with the poignant parental interviews of O'Moore (1978). Koegel et al. (1992) found that compared to the normative group on a test of resources and stress, mothers of children with autism from different cultural and geographic areas reported a characteristic pattern of worry about the child's dependency and long-term future.

Research results have been mixed as to the effect of the child's age on parental distress. Some studies found various indications that younger children are more difficult to parent (Bebko et al., 1987; Dumas et al., 1991; Gray & Holden, 1992), but others found that older children are more stressful (Bristol, 1984; Holroyd, Brown, Wikler, & Simmons, 1975; Konstantareas & Homatidis, 1989) or found no significant difference based on the child's age (Koegel et al., 1992). There are indications that mothers tend to experience distress earlier in the child's life than fathers do, perhaps as a combination of childcare demands and earlier awareness of the child's impairments (Bebko et al., 1987; Dumas et al., 1991).

Some studies found that the severity of the child's impairment was related to family stress (Bebko et al., 1987; Freeman, Perry, & Factor, 1991; Henderson & Vandenberg, 1992; Konstantareas & Homatidis, 1989; Konstantareas et al., 1992) but other studies have not found this association (Holroyd et al., 1975; Koegel et al., 1992; Milgrim & Atzil, 1988). One study even found that increased severity was associated with *less* marital stress, perhaps because severe disabilities are less ambiguous therefore less likely to lead to parental disagreement (Bristol, 1987).

It is generally accepted that factors such as social support and parents' coping strategies and belief systems play an important role in buffering parents from the stress of having a child with a disability (Bristol, 1987; Bristol, Gallagher, & Schopler, 1988; Henderson & Vandenberg, 1992; Sivberg, 1999; Tunali & Power, 2002; Weiss, 2002; Wolf, Noh, Fisman, & Speechley, 1989). Recognizing and responding to maternal distress is particularly important, since Robbins, Dunlap, and Plienis (1991) found that there was a significant negative correlation between mothers' stress levels and children's developmental progress in a parent training program. That is, the children of highly stressed mothers made less progress than the children of less stressed mothers.

Practical information also plays an important role in reducing parents' stress. Albanese, San Miguel, and Koegel (1995) reported that the families they worked with frequently requested and appreciated the following types of information: 1) a baby-sitter list; 2) a resource list of books, local professionals, national groups, etc. 3) contact information of other parents; 4) information on estate planning; and 5) advocacy resources.

Are There Commonalities Among Autism Parents?

Social Class

Based on Kanner's early observations about the intelligence and educational level of autism parents, for a time the professional community believed that autism was a disorder exclusively of highly educated, professional families. In fact, in describing early studies of the relationship of social class and autism, Schopler, Andrews, and Strupp (1979) wrote that "in some reports the higher social class status of parents was used as a *diagnostic selector* [emphasis added] for the child's inclusion in the autistic group" (p. 140).

However, the notion that autism occurs only in highly educated families was soon dispelled by both clinical experience and empirical research, as autism was found at all levels of socioeconomic status (SES; Gillberg & Schaumann, 1982; Ritvo et al., 1971; Schopler et al., 1979). Nevertheless, in a number of clinical samples of youngsters with autism (that is, youngsters identified through the clinical or educational services they received), the percentage of parents in the upper social classes was somewhat higher than the percentage of non-autism parents in those social classes (Bolton et al., 1994; Cantwell, Baker, & Rutter, 1979; Cox, Rutter, Newman, & Bartak, 1975; DeMyer, 1979; Eisenberg & Kanner, 1956; Kolvin, Ounsted, Richardson, & Garside, 1971; Rimland, 1964; Rutter & Lockyer, 1967; Sauna, 1987; Tsai, Stewart, Faust, & Shook, 1982).

Schopler et al. (1979) identified several factors that could account for the over-representation of higher SES families in clinical samples of autism. These factors included these parents' earlier recognition of developmental problems and greater ability to provide detailed the developmental history needed for a diagnosis of autism, and the ability of higher SES families to pay for and travel to services. Tsai et al. (1982) similarly concluded that when autism services were well-known and easily accessible, the overall distribution of social class of autism parents in their program was not significantly different from the distribution of social class in clinical control groups or the general population.

In contrast to clinical samples that are subject to various sociological factors that may bias results, epidemiological (or population) studies screen the population of a specified geographic area, and then study all subjects with the disorder. Wing (1980) reported that she and colleagues had not found evidence of an association between social class and autism in an epidemiologic study near London, and that a Danish researcher, Birte Hoeg Brask (Brask, 1972 as cited in Wing, 1980) had not found such an association in a similar study in a region of Denmark. However, Wing acknowledged that she was not able to explain the results of a landmark epidemiological study by Lotter (1967), who actually administered two intelligence tests to parents of children with autism identified through population screening in an English county and also compared the fathers' occupations to national norms. Lotter found that the autism parents as a group were markedly superior to the general population on both intelligence tests, and that the autism mothers, as a group, had higher intelligence than mothers of the control group of children without autism, even when social class and education were taken into account. In terms of fathers' occupations, in Lotter's sample of children with the most pronounced features of autism (marked social aloofness and repetitive/ritualistic behavior), 60% of the fathers were in the top 2 (of 5) social classes, compared with 24% of fathers of children with handicaps other than autism and with 23% of men in the general population. According to Wing, "the conclusion must be that Kanner's original observation of a very marked association between autism and high social class was at least partly due to selection factors, but it is not yet clear if there is some significant connection [between autism and socioeconomic status]" (Wing, 1980, p. 417).

Other epidemiological or quasi-epidemiological studies have also reported higher levels of paternal education (Treffert, 1970), paternal occupation (Steinhausen, Göbel, Breinlinger, & Wohlleben, 1986), or maternal education (Croen, Grether, Hoogstrate, & Selvin, 2002).

Although the issue of a possible slight over-representation of high SES or high intelligence among groups of autism parents periodically reappears and may be of interest to researchers, in clinical practice it is not particularly relevant. Autism spectrum disorders are found at all socioeconomic levels and in every country in which they have been sought (Discussions of ASD in other countries can be found in Cohen and Volkmar, 1997 and Schopler, 2000.)

Psychological Profiles

Before looking at the question of commonalities in the psychological profiles of parents, two important points must be made. First, the speculation that parents' personalities or behavior cause ASD was thoroughly discredited many years ago (Cantwell, Baker, & Rutter, 1978). Second, it is important to emphasize that patterns of personality *traits* are not the same as psychiatric *disorders*. Psychiatric disorders represent patterns of thinking, feeling, or behaving that are disruptive to some aspect of daily functioning (such as work, social, or family life) and that are unusual or uncommon. On the other hand, all human beings have patterns of personality characteristics, which psychologists have for years attempted to measure and categorize into meaningful patterns or traits.

In terms of psychiatric disorders, a few reports of psychological tests administered to autism parents in the 1970's and 1980's indicated no significant findings on self-report measures of psychopathology or personality such as the MMPI (Minnesota Multiphasic Personality Inventory), the Eysenck Personality Inventory, or the Maudsley Personality Inventory (Cantwell, Baker, & Rutter, 1979; DeMyer, 1979, Koegel, Schreibman, O'Neill, & Burke, 1983; Kolvin, Garside, & Kidd, 1971; McAdoo & DeMyer, 1978; Netley, Lockyer, & Greenbaum, 1975). However, a variety of studies using self-report measures of various symptoms of depression and anxiety found increased reports of psychological distress in autism parents (especially mothers) compared to parents of typical children, those with Down syndrome, or other clinical groups (Bristol,

Gallagher, & Schopler, 1988; DeMyer, 1979; Dumas et al., 1991; Gray & Holden, 1992; Milgrim & Atzil, 1988; Moes, Koegel, Schreibman, & Loos, 1992; Sharpley, Bitsika, & Efremidis, 1997; Weiss, 2002; Wolf et al., 1989).

Further, researchers at TEACCH and elsewhere have recently documented increased rates among autism parents of clinical depression compared to Down syndrome parents (Bolton, Pickles, Murphy, & Rutter, 1998; Piven et al., 1991; Piven & Palmer, 1999; Smalley et al., 1995). Earlier researchers tended to assume that parental depression resulted from the stress of caring for a child with autism, but these studies of four different samples of autism parents have documented that in the majority of cases of major depression, episodes of the disorder had occurred *before* the birth of the child with autism.

These studies also found increased rates in autism parents, compared to Down syndrome parents, of various anxiety disorders (Piven et al., 1991) and social phobia (Piven & Palmer, 1999; Smalley et al., 1995), and some indications of increased incidence of obsessive-compulsive disorder in the extended families (Bolton et al., 1998).

Piven (1999) has suggested several possible explanations for the finding of increased rates of depression among autism parents: 1) there is a genetic predisposition to depression in individuals who later produce a child with autism, or 2) individuals who are depressed or anxious have an increased incidence of marrying/having children with a partner who is genetically predisposed to produce a child with autism. At this time, the genetics of autism spectrum disorders are not yet clear, and research is ongoing.

Turning to the question of common personality traits, various researchers have for many years suggested that some parents (and other family members) may have milder or qualitatively similar forms of some of the behavioral characteristics that in their severe, combined form are called autism (Cantwell, Baker, & Rutter 1979; Eisenberg & Kanner, 1956; Narayan, Moyes, & Wolff, 1990; Netley et al., 1975). Conceptualizations used recently to describe these behavioral characteristics include a "lesser variant" of autism (Bolton et al., 1994) and the "Broader Autism Phenotype" (BAP; Piven, 1999). The theory underlying the concept of BAP is that several genes together produce the full-blown syndrome of an autism spectrum disorder, but when only some of these genes are present, the result may be certain qualitatively similar characteristics in a much milder form (Piven, 1999).

Research evidence for various dimensions of the BAP is growing (Fombonne, Bolton, Prior, Jordan, & Murphy, 1997; Murphy et al., 2000; Piven, 1999; Piven, Palmer, Jacobi, Childress, & Arndt, 1997). Several studies have found subtle language difficulties among autism parents. Landa, Folstein, and Isaacs (1991) reported that a subgroup (34%) of autism parents in their sample had significant difficulty with generating a complete, coherent children's story on request, and several other parents refused to attempt the task, saying it was too difficult. Landa et al. (1992) found that a subgroup (42%) of autism parents in their sample had mild, non-impairing, but still measurable difficulties with various aspects of social and pragmatic language (that is, the ability to use language fluidly in socially appropriate and effective ways). Folstein et al. (1999)

identified a subgroup (24%) of autism parents who as children had language-related difficulties, and as adults had mild difficulties with various language-based cognitive tasks, such as spelling and phonics/word attack skills. Slightly different results were reported by Piven and Palmer (1997) in a different sample of autism parents: as a group these parents did not have difficulty with spelling or simple reading/decoding, but they did show deficits in rapid word-finding and reading comprehension compared to a group of Down Syndrome parents. (This study reported only overall group findings and did not indicate whether these results were found only in a subgroup of parents.)

Other research on parental commonalities has looked at issues of social awkwardness and stereotyped or rigid behaviors. Using a standardized personality interview, Piven et al. (1994) reported that the autism parents rated themselves as significantly more 'aloof', 'untactful', and 'unresponsive' to the social-emotional cues of others, than did a control group of Down Syndrome parents on the same measures. Piven, Palmer, Landa et al. (1997), with a different sample of autism parents, replicated many of these findings using 'best estimates' of personality traits based on evaluations of both self-reports and reports from spouses, and also found significantly elevated ratings on 'rigidity,' defined as both difficulty with change and limited interest in new situations or ideas.

Another commonality among autism parents identified by several research groups is in the area of executive function. "Executive Function" refers to a variety of cognitive activities such as planning, organizing, shifting focus as needed, inhibiting automatic responses, and memory. Hughes, Leboyer, and Bouvard (1997) reported the results of three executive function tests with autism parents, parents of children with mental retardation, and typical adults. As a group, the autism parents made significantly more errors than the other groups on tasks involving shifting attention, planning, and working memory, while not showing significant differences on other, non-executive function tasks (discrimination learning, spatial memory). Also, there was a correlation for autism parents as a group between their overall executive function score and pre-testing descriptions of their social behaviors (more difficulty with executive functions was associated with more unusual social behavior). On further analysis, the difficulties with executive function were found to occur predominantly in a subgroup of 25% of the autism parents. A deficit among autism parents relative to controls was also reported by Piven and Palmer (1997) on a standard executive function/planning task (Tower of Hanoi).

In summary, the research and clinical literature in the area of parents has moved away from the initial theory that parents cause autism, through a period in which autism parents were thought to be indistinguishable from other parents except for child-induced stress, to current thinking that autism parents as a group have increased rates of apparently biologically-based depression, anxiety, and some aspects of executive functions, and that *some* autism parents also demonstrate *some* isolated characteristics qualitatively similar to autism spectrum disorders in a much milder form.

PARENT TRAINING PROGRAMS

The co-founders of the TEACCH program were among the first professionals to suggest that parents could learn to work as 'co-therapists' for their children (Schopler & Reichler, 1971), and none of the evidence about parental characteristics just cited would argue against that. TEACCH research has confirmed that autism parents can be very effective in teaching their children a variety of skills (Marcus, Lansing, Andrews, & Schopler, 1978; Schopler, Mesibov, & Baker, 1982; Short, 1984). Some researchers have even reported that parents are *more effective* at teaching than clinic-based therapists (Koegel et al., 1982; Schopler & Reichler, 1971). Dawson and Osterling (1997) reported that parent training was a component of all the successful early intervention programs they identified for children with autism. Further, there are indications that parent training contributes to reducing mothers' depressive symptoms (Bristol, Gallagher, & Holt, 1993) and increasing positive family interactions (Koegel, Bimbela & Schreibman, 1996; Moes, 1995) and recreational activities (Koegel et al., 1982).

Traditional Behavioral Methods

One model of parent training has been teaching parents standard operant learning procedures such as cueing, prompting, positively reinforcing, and extinguishing behavior. An early study using these techniques was carried out by Lovaas, Koegel, Simmons, and Long (1973), who reported on a series of 13 children with autism who had learned new skills in either an inpatient or outpatient behavior therapy setting. After the operant learning treatment, some children went on to custodial institutions or other residential settings where behavioral methods were not used. On follow-up four years later, these children had lost most of the skills they had learned. However, the treated children whose parents had also been trained in the behavioral methods maintained some skills, or in some cases continued to make progress. (Although this study is often cited as demonstrating the importance of parent training in behavioral methods, there was no control group of children who were treated then went home for similar periods of time to parents who had *not* been trained, so the interpretability of this study in terms of the importance of parent *training* is limited.)

A more recent report of parent training (Smith, Groen, & Wynn, 2000, 2001) involved subjects from Lovaas' UCLA Young Autism Project. Twenty-eight children (mean age 3 years) were assigned either to parent training in behavioral techniques (two home visits totaling five hours per week for 3–9 months) or to intensive behavioral treatment from 4–6 student therapists (averaging 24.5 hours per week for at least 18 months). On follow-up assessment (mean age 7 years, 7–8 months) the authors reported that the intensive treatment group scored higher than the parent training group on an IQ test (although both groups remained significantly delayed) and on visual-spatial skills and some aspects of language.

Although behavioral parent training programs have generally reported good success initially, several follow-up studies have found that many parents eventually discontinued using the operant learning procedures in which they had been trained (Harris & Powers, 1984). For example, Howlin, Rutter, and colleagues (Howlin & Rutter, 1987) developed a comprehensive, home-based program in which parents of children with autism, aged 2–11 years, were taught operant learning techniques by clinical psychologists, with the goals of stimulating the children's communication, play, and social skill development. (The psychologists also provided emotional and logistical support for the families, so the scope of the project was broader than just teaching behavioral methods.) Training was provided during home visits (at least weekly visits for approximately 6 months, then generally tapered to 2–3 times a month for 6 months, then to once a month for the final 6 months). The study involved 16 families, who were compared on a number of variables after the training program to matched control groups who did not receive the same treatment and intensity. At the end of 18 months, the children in the treatment group were more improved than the control groups in social communication, cooperation, and play patterns, and they also displayed less ritualistic behavior and fewer tantrums. However, in a follow-up study of the families in this study, Holmes, Helmsley, Rickett, and Likierman (1982) wrote that "few parents [in the parent training group] reported that they were still using the techniques, and, in fact, there were no differences between the [experimental and control] groups in their perceptions of general improvement after help had ended. Both groups felt that things had improved or stayed the same" (p. 340–341).

Harris, Wolchik, and Weitz (1981) taught parents of preschool children with autism the principles of behavior modification and operant speech training during a 10-week group workshop. Most of the children made progress on a hierarchy of language skills during the program, but at 1-year follow up most had not made further progress. The researchers observed that most families no longer engaged in formal teaching sessions. Later research (Harris, 1986) confirmed this observation: 56% of the families studied reported that they had not "used formal behavior modification procedures including data collection to teach ... [the] child a new skill or control a behavior problem" in the past year (p. 42). However, 86% had used some elements of behavior modification to manage their children's behavior in the past week, and 58% had used some element of behavior modification to teach their child a new skill during that time. The fathers' use of the techniques seemed to be dependent on the mothers' use of them, and both parents were more likely to use them if school personnel did so.

Koegel et al. (1982) reported results of a project in which children with autism, aged 2–10 years, were randomly assigned to either parent training or clinic-based behavioral treatment. Parents were rigorously trained to criterion in operant learning principles and techniques, after which they received monthly home visits and access to telephone consultation for a year. The clinic-based treatment consisted of the same behavior modification that the parents learned, administered by trained staff. At the end of the year, children in both groups showed improvements in appropriate behavior with their treatment provider, but only children in the parent training condition showed improvement with their mothers. Children in the parent training group also showed improvements relative to the clinic-based group during unstructured observation at home. Neither group showed significant improvement with a stranger. In describing the same project, Schreibman, Koegel, Mills, and Burke (1984) reported that the trained parents reported a *decrease* in their self-appraisal of their ability to work with their own children (although this may have been due to their overestimating their skills before training). Further, 62% of parents who had received both the parent training and clinic-based services (at different times, in random order across the sample) indicated that they preferred the clinic-based services. However, this preference may have been attributable to the fact that the clinic-based services were free. When the parents were asked the same question with a substantial hourly fee attached to the clinic-based services, 92% preferred a combination of parent training and clinic-based treatment for the child.

Modern Behavioral Methods

In 1986, Helm and Kozloff suggested that the behavioral parent training programs they reviewed reflected an inadequate model of human behavior and development, focused too heavily on isolated behaviors rather than a flexible, functional repertoire of skills, and failed to evaluate outcome issues such as improvements in parents' self-concepts and in family dynamics.

Along these lines, Koegel and Schreibman, who earlier had pioneered work in teaching operant learning techniques (e.g., Koegel et al., 1982), came to realize the limitations of these techniques for students with autism. In a typical operant learning procedure, the adult sets up a discrete learning trial by giving a direction, then rewards the child for a pre-defined correct response with food or praise. Koegel and Schreibman developed an alternative technique they called "pivotal response training" (Schreibman, 1997) which includes, among other features, following the child's lead in choosing objects to play with or talk about, rewarding all of the child's attempts to respond, and using natural reinforcers (such as giving the child the toy car he wants if he attempts to say "car"). Koegel et al. (1996) reported results of a study in which two groups of autism parents were randomly assigned to either the standard discrete trial training or pivotal response training. After the families had mastered their teaching techniques, they were compared on various dimensions. The families in the pivotal response group were significantly happier, less stressed, more engaged in interacting with their children, and more positive in their communication style than the parents in the discrete trial training group.

Similarly, Koegel, Symon, and Koegel (2002) described a clinical study in which families of children with autism were taught pivotal response techniques during an intensive 5-day program. Analysis of videotapes recorded at home at least three months after the intervention program indicated that all the parents continued to use the techniques correctly, all of the children's functional expressive language increased compared to baseline, and all the parents were rated by observers as interacting more positively with their children compared to pre-intervention levels. Kaiser, Hancock, and Nietfeld (2000) demonstrated that parents could learn to implement "enhanced milieu teaching" (a naturalistic language intervention approach similar to pivotal response training), which resulted in positive changes and long-term (6 months) maintenance of most children's social communication after the parent training had ended, as well as high parental satisfaction with the approach.

Several authors have emphasized that although it is important for parents to learn specific teaching techniques (Harris, Wochik, & Milch, 1982), also learning general principles seems likely to have longer-term benefits (Helm & Kozloff, 1986; Holmes et al., 1982; Moes, 1995; Schreibman et al., 1984). This position is related to evidence indicating that empowering parents to individualize the application of behavioral principles to their particular family situation is desirable. For example, Frea and Hepburn (1999) demonstrated in a pilot study that two parents benefited from learning assessment and analytic skills then designing their own interventions, teaching functional equivalents of difficult behaviors (such as saying "help me" instead of becoming aggressive or self-injurious). Stiebel (1999) reported that children's spontaneous communication generalized to additional settings when parents were taught a problem-solving process to analyze how to make additional communication opportunities available in ways that the parents determined were comfortable and consistent with their lifestyle. Moes and Frea (2002) reported on a study in which "information on family context was used to individualize behavioral support plans designed to support family use of functional communication training within important family routines" (p. 519) and that "consideration of family context in the assessment and intervention planning process does not jeopardize and may contribute to the stability and durability of reductions in challenging behavior" (p. 519). Similarly, Marshall and Mirenda (2002) stressed the importance of working collaboratively with parents, rather than simply designing a behavior management plan. In the case study they presented, the process of collaboration between parent and professionals yielded a practical behavior support plan that both parents agreed with, and that gave the parents practice and confidence in applying analytic and therapeutic techniques, so that they were better-prepared to handle new problems in the future.

Related to programs of teaching general principles of intervention are psychoeducational programs designed to help parents understand ASD. Shields (2001) described the EarlyBird Programme developed by the National Autistic Society (United Kingdom), which begins with providing information about ASD before introducing specific skills for stimulating communication and managing behavior; preliminary results of this program are encouraging and a formal efficacy study is ongoing. Sofronoff and Farbotko (2002) demonstrated that a psychoeducational program designed to help parents understand the perspective of their child with Asperger syndrome resulted in a decrease in the number of reported behavior problems. Concepts taught in this psychoeducational program included the nature of Asperger syndrome, techniques such as Comic

Strip Conversations and Social Stories (Gray, 1998) to assist children with understanding social situations, and the characteristics of Asperger Syndrome that
underlie problem behaviors and anxiety. The program was in some ways more
effective for mothers than for fathers, and the authors observed that several
of the fathers in their study "displayed traits of Asperger Syndrome" (p. 281)
which might have reduced the benefits they obtained from an orally-presented
psychoeducational program. The authors suggested that more visually-based or
experiential training might have been more effective for these fathers.

Multi-faceted Programs for Parents

Recent work in parent education has focused more broadly than teaching standard behavioral techniques and principles, similar in some ways to
the classic work of Howlin and Rutter (1987), which included parent support
along with teaching strategies. For example, Harris (1984a, 1984b) has long ad-
vocated that clinicians attend both to the behavior management skills and to
the emotional health of individual family members and the family system, in
order to develop effective individualized intervention programs. Konstantareas
(1990) has summarized a comprehensive psychoeducational approach to work
with family members that both addresses their grief and psychological needs,
and provides practical recommendations about developmental stimulation and
child management. Whitaker (2002) reported that many parents wanted help in
supporting other areas of their child's development in addition to addressing
the characteristics of autism.

Studies supporting the value of various facets of parent programs include
that by Stahmer and Gist (2001), in which one group of autism parents received
only individualized skill training, while the other group received that training but also attended a parent education support group. Results were striking
in showing both the importance of the parent group for mastering teaching
skills, and the importance of those teaching skills for child progress. Bitsika
and Sharpley (1999, 2000) found that teaching mothers specific behavioral stress
management techniques (such as deep breathing, progressive muscle relaxation,
and biofeedback) was rated by most mothers as the most valuable element of
a multi-faceted parent support group. Whitaker (2002) interviewed parents of
preschool children who had received services from a multi-faceted autism support program, and found that both practical information (e.g., information about
ASD and strategies for managing and teaching their children) and emotional
support were highly valued by parents.

Other Issues in Parent Training

Several researchers have found that there are sub-groups of parents who
have not benefited from available parent training programs (Symon, 2001).
Helm and Kozloff (1986) wrote that their research indicated that "approximately one-third of the families thrive on such programs, one-third are helped

to a more limited extent, and one-third are not appreciably changed during the program" (p. 16–17). Similarly, Plienis, Robbins, and Dunlap (1988) wrote that "We have clearly seen a wide range of responses to training, with some families that do extremely well while others respond less successfully. The data presented on the efficacy of major parent training projects are typically presented in a grouped fashion which can mask a considerable range of individual differences or the presence of sub-group outliers" (p. 35). Whitaker (2002) noted that when parent training was provided shortly after the child was diagnosed, some parents were not emotionally ready to take in the information and apply it. He also reported that in the families who chose not to participate in the training program, "the main wage earner has tended to be in less well paid or secure employment, there has often been another very young infant, and the families have often appeared to be struggling with a range of demands on their organizational abilities" (p. 418).

Summary

The modern clinical and research literature related to autism parents supports the following conclusions:

- Parents of youngsters with autism experience increased logistical demands and stress relative to parents of other youngsters, and they have increased rates of depression and anxiety. Further, some parents themselves have personality characteristics related to autism (Piven, 1999).
- Social, emotional, and practical support provide buffers that reduce some of the distress that parents experience. No one approach is helpful to all parents. Some parents need very explicit, written information and hands-on practice, not just verbal discussions of their child's needs.
- Parents value practical information and guidance in understanding their child's autism, learning specific teaching techniques, and learning general principles to apply to new skills and situations.

TEACCH's WORK WITH FAMILIES

The TEACCH approach to working with parents follows the research literature about the elements of professional interventions that are important for parents, specifically:

- Teaching parents to understand the nature of autism spectrum disorders
- Providing both specific strategies and general approaches to skill development and behavior management
- Identifying and facilitating individualized interventions for each family
- Introducing parents to a supportive, welcoming network of professionals and other parents who understand and appreciate ASD and the difficulties families often face (Marcus, 1977).

Values

In providing these services, the fundamental value of the TEACCH approach to parents is respect.

- TEACCH respects parents' *knowledge* of their child, recognizing that while professionals have a wide range of knowledge about children with special needs, parents know their own child better than anyone else, and recognizing that the limited observations of professionals in clinical settings must be supplemented by the rich and often more comprehensive observations made by parents.
- TEACCH respects the *individuality* of each family, knowing that their priorities should guide all work with them, and that as much as possible work should be at a tempo that is comfortable for them (although limited resources and great demand sometimes mean that we must ration our services and arrange appointments on an organized, predictable schedule). The wide range of parents' backgrounds, personalities, needs, and talents can be accommodated within this framework of respect for individuality.
- TEACCH respects the *love* that parents have for their children, being their most passionate and dedicated caregivers and advocates long after professionals have moved on to other positions, agencies, or activities.
- TEACCH respects the *resilience* of parents in finding solutions and ways of coping that work best for them and their families, in the face of intense needs and stresses (Schopler, 1995).
- TEACCH respects the *contributions* parents make through political advocacy, developing new services, and volunteering their time to help and support other families.
- TEACCH respects the *needs* of parents for accurate information, emotional support, comprehensive services, and professional guidance in teaching their child skills for becoming as independent as possible.

Organization of Services

The TEACCH program has grown in size and geographic location over the years. Because of the differing characteristics of the various areas of North Carolina in which the 9 TEACCH Centers are located, and because of the unique skills and visions of TEACCH professionals in each Center, specific clinical activities within TEACCH vary more now than they did in earlier years when TEACCH consisted of 3–5 centers (Schopler, Mesibov, Shigley, and Bashford, 1984) but in all centers, work with parents is based on the elements of respect just described and on our core values (see Chapter 2, Core Values of TEACCH).

The initial referral to a TEACCH Center can be made by a parent or by a professional, advocate, or other support person. If parents are seeking a diagnostic evaluation, we request that they arrange for TEACCH to receive any prior evaluation reports, and we ask for their perspectives on their child's skills and needs.

One method of obtaining valuable parental input is asking them to write a description, of whatever length they choose, of a typical day with their youngster. During the diagnostic evaluation (which typically takes during one day-long session, although this can be modified as needed) parents are interviewed in depth about their child's skills, behaviors, and needs, but are also invited to watch part of the testing session with the child (or sometimes to participate in that session, if the child needs to have the parent present) so that they can feel comfortable about the child's well-being, and also so that they can give the TEACCH professionals feedback about whether we are getting a valid picture of the child's skills and behavior. After a staff conference in which all the diagnostic information is integrated, the Clinical Director (a doctoral level psychologist) and other evaluation staff meet with the parents to answer their questions, provide information about diagnosis and recommendations, and support them as they receive the diagnostic results. (See Chapter 9, Providing Diagnostic Information to Parents, for additional information about interpretive sessions.) The youngster's diagnostic report is written for parents to read and distribute to other professionals and agencies as they choose.

In recent years, more and more families come to TEACCH Centers having already received the diagnosis of an autism spectrum disorder from other professionals. We have therefore developed mechanisms for these families to by-pass the waiting list for diagnostic evaluations and enter directly into treatment services. These services used to be called the "extended diagnostic" but are now also referred to as "teaching sessions," "treatment sessions," or "parent education sessions."

Typically, two psychoeducational therapists work together with each family, one therapist taking the role of "Parent Consultant" while the other is called the "Child Therapist" (although services are provided to individuals of all ages). All therapists take on both roles within each Center. The first treatment session is generally a meeting of the two therapists with the parents to establish needs and goals; sometimes the Clinical Director also participates in this session. Typically then 6–8 hourly sessions are scheduled to work on these goals. Sessions are usually held weekly or every other week, although appointments can be individualized as needed. TEACCH diagnostic and treatment services are free to residents of North Carolina. Because of the enormous demand on TEACCH's limited resources, standard treatment services are generally limited to eight sessions, but parents are assured that TEACCH remains available to them indefinitely for consultation and urgent needs.

Useful Treatment Strategies

Treatment services provided take many forms. A recent survey of the types of services that have been provided to parents within the 9 TEACCH Centers yielded the following list:

- Demonstrations by a therapist of working with the individual on various skill-building activities (such as cognitive, visual-motor, language/communication, independent play, and self-help skills), and demonstrations by the parent with feedback from the therapist. All TEACCH Centers are equipped with one-way mirrors and sound systems so that parents can observe the youngster working with a therapist, and vice versa.

- Demonstrations of the use of picture and/or written schedules for making transitions between activities
- Videotapes of these demonstrations for parents to review at home or share with other family members
- Written home programs focused on skill development
- Discussions of the nature of autism (see Chapter 3, The Culture of Autism) and the application in the home of Structured Teaching principles (see Chapter 4, Structured Teaching)
- "Make and Take" sessions in which parents and therapists together prepare materials for use at home
- Suggested readings and websites
- Home visits to address issues of physical structure (see Chapter 4, Structured Teaching) and/or to demonstrate working with the child in the home setting
- Suggested 'homework' and/or data collection systems for use at home
- Individual sessions with a parent to provide support and referrals for other needed services
- Family counseling sessions with parents and their adolescent/adult children with High Functioning Autism/Asperger Syndrome
- Workshops for parents on topics such as Structured Teaching, Writing Social Stories (Gray, 1998), and High Functioning Autism/Asperger Syndrome. Parents are also welcome to attend other TEACCH training programs designed for teachers and other professionals
- Facilitation of parent support groups, which have included mothers' groups, fathers' groups, groups for parents of adults with ASD, and groups for parents of youngsters who are participating in social groups at the same time.
- Professional presentations at parent groups
- Attendance at school IEP and other agency meetings with parents

Parent Satisfaction

As part of ongoing program evaluation of TEACCH services, we asked parents who received diagnostic and/or treatment services from several of the regional TEACCH centers during the past 1–2 years for feedback about various aspects of the services they had received. Fifty-eight parents responded, and on a scale of 1 (very dissatisfied) to 5 (very satisfied), their average responses on selected items were as follows:

Evaluations

- The results of the TEACCH evaluation were clearly and fully explained   **4.91**

- Your questions and concerns about your child were clearly addressed   **4.90**
- Overall, you were satisfied with the TEACCH evaluation   **4.85**

  Treatment Sessions

- The treatment sessions focused on the concerns and problems that you identified during your initial meeting   **4.85**
- You found these strategies helpful when you used them at home or in other settings   **4.83**
- Overall you were satisfied with the TEACCH individualized family treatment sessions   **4.85**

CONCLUDING COMMENTS

The principles of understanding the culture of autism, individualized assessment and treatment, and respect for parents have been the foundation of the TEACCH program for over 30 years (Marcus, Kunce, and Schopler, 1997). We work with each individual family according to their needs, strengths, resources, challenges, and preferences. Consistent with the research literature, we have found that a flexible, multi-faceted approach to sharing our expertise in autism is both effective and appreciated by parents.

REFERENCES

Albanese, A.L., San Miguel, S.E., & Koegel, R.L. (1995). Social support for families. In R.L. Koegel & L.K. Koegel (Eds.), *Teaching children with autism: Strategies for initiating positive interactions and improving learning opportunities* (pp. 95–104). Baltimore: Paul Brookes.

Bebko, J.M., Konstantareas, M.M., & Springer, J. (1987). Parent and professional evaluations of family stress associated with characteristics of autism. *Journal of Autism and Developmental Disorders, 17,* 565–576.

Bettelheim, B. (1967). *The empty fortress: Infantile autism and the birth of the self.* New York: Free Press.

Bitseka, V. & Sharpley, C. (1999). An exploratory examination of the effects of support groups on the well-being of parents of children with autism—I: General counseling. *Journal of Applied Health Behavior, 1,* 16–22.

Bitseka, V. & Sharpley, C. (2000). Development and testing of the effects of support groups on the well-being of parents of children with autism—II: Specific stress management techniques. *Journal of Applied Health Behavior, 2,* 8–15.

Bolton, P., Macdonald, A., Pickles, A., Rios., P., Goode, S., Crowson, M. et al. (1994). A case-control family history study of autism. *Journal of Child Psychology and Psychiatry, 35,* 877–900.

Bolton, P.F., Pickles, A., Murphy, M., & Rutter, M. (1998). Autism, affective and other psychiatric disorders: Patterns of familial aggregation. *Psychological Medicine, 28,* 385–395.

Bouma, R. & Schweitzer, R. (1990). The impact of chronic childhood illness on family stress: A comparison between autism and cystic fibrosis. *Journal of Clinical Psychology, 46,* 722–730.

Bristol, M.M. (1984) Family resources and successful adaptation to autistic children. In E. Schopler & G.B Mesibov (Eds.), *The effects of autism on the family* (pp. 289–310). New York: Plenum Press.

Bristol, M.M. (1987). Mothers of children with autism or communication disorders: Successful adaptation and the Double ABCX model. *Journal of Autism and Developmental Disorders, 17,* 469–486.

Bristol, M.M. Gallagher, J.J., & Holt, K.D. (1993). Maternal depressive symptoms in autism: Response to psychoeducational intervention. *Rehabilitation Psychology, 38,* 3–10.

Bristol, M.M., Gallagher, J.J., & Schopler, E. (1988). Mothers and fathers of young developmentally disabled and nondisabled boys: Adaptation and spousal support. *Developmental Psychology, 24,* 441–451.

Cantwell, D.P., Baker, L., & Rutter, M. (1978). Family factors. In M. Rutter & E. Schopler (Eds.), *Autism: A reappraisal of concepts and treatment* (pp. 269–296). New York: Plenum Press.

Cantwell, D.P., Baker, L., & Rutter, M. (1979). Families of autistic and dysphasic children—I. Family life and interaction patterns. *Archives of General Psychiatry, 36,* 682–688.

Cohen, D.J. & Volkmar, F.R. (Eds.). (1997). *Handbook of autism and pervasive developmental disorders.* New York: John Wiley & Sons.

Cox, A., Rutter, M., Newman, S., & Bartak, L. (1975). A comparative study of infantile autism and specific developmental receptive language disorder: II. Parental characteristics. *British Journal of Psychiatry, 126,* 146–159.

Croen, L.A., Grether, J.K., Hoogstrate, J., & Selvin, S. (2002). Descriptive epidemiology of autism in a California population: Who is at risk? *Journal of Autism and Developmental Disorders, 32,* 217–224.

Dawson, G. & Osterling, J. (1997). Early intervention in autism. In M.J. Guralnick (Ed.), *The effectiveness of early intervention.* (pp. 307–326). Baltimore: Paul Brookes.

DeMyer, M.K. (1979). *Parents and children in autism.* New York: John Wiley & Sons.

DeMyer, M.K. & Goldberg, P. (1983). Family needs of the autistic adolescent. In E. Schopler & G. B Mesibov (Eds.), *Autism in adolescents and adults* (pp. 225–250). New York: Plenum Press.

Dumas, J.E., Wolf, L.C., Fisman, S.N., & Culligan, A. (1991). Parenting stress, child behavior problems, and dysphoria in parents of children with autism, Down syndrome, behavior disorders, and normal development. *Exceptionality, 2,* 97–110.

Eisenberg, L. & Kanner, L. (1956). Early infantile autism, 1943–55. *American Journal of Orthopsychiatry, 26,* 556–566.

Fisman, S.N., Wolf, L.C., & Noh, S. (1989). Marital intimacy in parents of exceptional children. *Canadian Journal of Psychiatry, 34,* 519–525.

Folstein, S.E., Santangelo, S.L., Gilman, S.E., Piven, J., Landa, R., Lainhart, J. et al. (1999). Predictors of cognitive test patterns in autism families. *Journal of Child Psychology & Psychiatry & Allied Disciplines, 40,* 1117–1128.

Fombonne, E., Bolton, P., Prior, J., Jordan, H., & Rutter, M. (1997). A family study of autism: Cognitive patterns and levels in parents and siblings. *Journal of Child Psychology & Psychiatry & Allied Disciplines, 38,* 667–683.

Fong, L., Wilgosh, L., & Sobsey, D. (1993). The experience of parenting an adolescent with autism. *International Journal of Disability, Development & Education, 40,* 105–113.

Frea, W.D. & Hepburn, S.L. (1999). Teaching parents of children with autism to perform functional assessments to plan interventions for extremely disruptive behaviors. *Journal of Positive Behavior Interventions, 1,* 112–116.

Freeman, N.L., Perry, A., & Factor, D.C. (1991). Child behaviors as stressors: Replicating and extending the use of the CARS as a measure of stress: A research note. *Journal of Child Psychology and Psychiatry, 32,* 1025–1030.

Gillberg, C. & Schaumann, H. (1982). Social class and infantile autism. *Journal of Autism and Developmental Disorders, 12,* 223–228.

Gray, C. (1998). Social stories and comic strip conversations with students with Asperger syndrome and high-functioning autism. In E. Schopler, G.B. Mesibov, & L.J. Kunce (Eds.), *Asperger syndrome or high-functioning autism?* (pp. 167–198). New York: Plenum Press.

Gray, D.E. & Holden, W.J. (1992). Psycho-social well-being among the parents of children with autism. *Australia & New Zealand Journal of Developmental Disabilities, 18,* 83–93.

Harris, S.L. (1984a). Intervention planning for the family of the autistic child: A multilevel assessment of the family system. *Journal of Marital and Family Therapy, 10,* 157–166.

Harris, S.L. (1984b). The family of the autistic child: A behavioral-systems view. *Clinical Psychology Review, 4,* 227–239.

Harris, S.L. (1986). Parents as teachers: A four to seven year follow up of parents of children with autism. *Child & Family Behavior Therapy, 8,* 39–47.

Harris, S.L. & Powers, M. (1984). Behavior therapists look at the impact of an autistic child on the family system. In E. Schopler & G. B Mesibov (Eds.), *The effects of autism on the family* (pp. 207–224). New York: Plenum Press.

Harris, S.L., Wolchik, S.A. & Milch, R.E. (1982). Changing the speech of autistic children and their parents. *Child & Family Behavior Therapy, 4,* 151–173.

Harris, S.L., Wolchik, S.A., & Weitz, S. (1981). The acquisition of language skills by autistic children: Can parents do the job? *Journal of Autism and Developmental Disorders, 11,* 373–384.

Helm, D.T. & Kozloff, M.A. (1986). Research on parent training: Shortcomings and remedies. *Journal of Autism and Developmental Disorders, 16,* 1–22.

Henderson, D. & Vandenberg, B. (1992). Factors influencing adjustment in the families of autistic children. *Psychological Reports, 71,* 167–171.

Holmes, N., Hemsley, R., Rickett, J., & Likierman, H. (1982). Parents as cotherapists: Their perceptions of a home-based behavioral treatment for autistic children. *Journal of Autism and Developmental Disorders, 12,* 331–342.

Holroyd, J., Brown, N., Wikler, L., & Simmons, J.Q. (1975). Stress in families of institutionalized and noninstitutionalized autistic children. *Journal of Community Psychology, 3,* 26–31.

Holroyd, J. & McArthur, D. (1976). Mental retardation and stress on the parents: A contrast between Down's syndrome and childhood autism. *American Journal of Mental Deficiency, 80,* 431–436.

Hoppes, K. & Harris, S.L. (1990). Perceptions of child attachment and maternal gratification in mothers of children with autism and Down syndrome. *Journal of Clinical Child Psychology, 19,* 365–370.

Howlin, P. & Rutter, M. (with Berger, M., Hemsley, R., Hersov, L., & Yule, W.). (1987). *Treatment of autistic children.* New York: John Wiley & Sons.

Hughes, C., Leboyer, M., & Bouvard, M. (1997). Executive function in parents of children with autism. *Psychological Medicine, 27,* 209–220.

Kaiser, A.P., Hancock, T.B., & Nietfeld, J.P. (2000). The effects of parent-implemented Enhanced Milieu Teaching on the social communication of children who have autism. *Early Education & Development, 11,* 423–446.

Kanner, L. (1943). Autistic disturbances of affective contact. *Nervous Child, 2,* 217–250.

Kanner, L. (1949). Problems of nosology and psychodynamics of early infantile autism. *American Journal of Orthopsychiatry, 19,* 416–426.

Kanner, L. (1968). Early infantile autism revisited. *Psychiatry Digest, 29,* 17–28.

Koegel, R.L., Bimbela, A., & Schreibman, L. (1996). Collateral effects of parent training on family interactions. *Journal of Autism and Developmental Disorders, 26,* 347–359.

Koegel, R.L., Schreibman, L., Britten, K.R., Burke, J.C., & O'Neill, R.E. (1982). A comparison of parent training to direct child treatment. In R.L. Koegel, A. Rincover, & A.L. Egel. *Educating and understanding autistic children.* (pp. 260–279). San Diego: College Hill Press.

Koegel, R.L., Schreibman, L., Loos, L.M., Dirlich-Wilhelm, H., Dunlap, G., Robbins, F.R., et al. (1992). Consistent stress profiles in mothers of children with autism. *Journal of Autism and Developmental Disorders, 22,* 205–216.

Koegel, R.L., Schreibman, L., O'Neill, R.E., & Burke, J.C. (1983). The personality and family-interaction characteristics of parents of autistic children. *Journal of Consulting & Clinical Psychology, 51,* 683–692.

Koegel, R.L., Symon, J.B., & Koegel, L.K. (2002). Parent education for families of children with autism living in geographically distant areas. *Journal of Positive Behavior Interventions, 4,* 88–103.

Kohler, F.W. (1999). Examining the services received by young children with autism and their families: A survey of parent responses. *Focus on Autism and other Developmental Disabilities, 14,* 150–158.

Kolvin, I., Garside, R.F., & Kidd, J.S.H. (1971). IV. Parental personality and attitude and childhood psychoses. *British Journal of Psychiatry, 118*, 403–406.

Kolvin, I., Ounsted, C., Richardson, L.M., & Garside, R.F. (1971). III. The family and social background in childhood psychoses. *British Journal of Psychiatry, 118*, 396–402.

Konstantareas, M.M. (1990). A psychoeducational model for working with families of autistic children. *Journal of Marital & Family Therapy, 16*, 59–70.

Konstantareas, M.M. & Homatidis, S. (1989). Assessing child symptom severity and stress in parents of autistic children. *Journal of Child Psychology & Psychiatry & Allied Disciplines, 30*, 459–470.

Konstantareas, M.M., Homatidis, S., & Plowright, C.M.S. (1992). Assessing resources and stress in parents of severely dysfunctional children through the Clarke modification of Holroyd's Questionnaire on Resources and Stress. *Journal of Autism and Developmental Disorders, 22*, 217–234.

Landa, R., Folstein, S.E., & Isaacs, C. (1991). Spontaneous narrative-discourse performance of parents of autistic individuals. *Journal of Speech & Hearing Research, 34*, 1339–1345.

Landa, R., Piven, J., Wzorek, M.M., Gayle, J.O., Chase, G.A., & Folstein, S. (1992). Social language use in parents of autistic individuals. *Psychological Medicine, 22*, 245–254.

Lotter, V. (1967). Epidemiology of autistic conditions in young children: II. Some characteristics of the parents and children. *Social Psychiatry, 1*, 163–173.

Lovaas, O.I., Koegel, R., Simmons, J.Q., & Long, J.S. (1973). Some generalization and follow-up measures on autistic children in behavior therapy. *Journal of Applied Behavior Analysis, 6*, 131–166.

Marcus, L.M. (1977). Patterns of coping in families of psychotic children. *American Journal of Orthopsychiatry, 47*, 388–399.

Marcus, L.M., Kunce, L.J., & Schopler, E. (1997). Working with families. In D.J. Cohen & F.R. Volkmar (Eds.), *Handbook of autism and pervasive developmental disorders* (pp. 631–649). New York: John Wiley & Sons.

Marcus, L.M., Lansing, M., Andrews, C.E., & Schopler, E. (1978). Improvement of teaching effectiveness in parents of autistic children. *Journal of the American Academy of Child Psychiatry 17*, 625–639.

Marshall, J.K. & Mirenda, P. (2002). Parent-professional collaboration for positive behavior support in the home. *Focus on Autism and Other Developmental Disabilities, 17*, 216–228.

McAdoo, W.G. & DeMyer, M.K. (1978). Personality characteristics of parents. In M. Rutter & E. Schopler (Eds.), *Autism: A reappraisal of concepts and treatment.* (pp. 251–267). New York: Plenum Press.

Midence, K. & O'Neill, M. (1999). The experience of parents in the diagnosis of autism. *Autism, 3*, 273–285.

Milgram, N.A. & Atzil, M. (1988). Parenting stress in raising autistic children. *Journal of Autism and Developmental Disorders, 18*, 415–424.

Moes, D.R. (1995). Parent education and parent stress. In R.L. Koegel & L.K. Koegel (Eds.), *Teaching children with autism: Strategies for initiating positive interact tions and improving learning opportunities* (pp. 79–93). Baltimore: Paul Brookes.

Moes, D.R. & Frea, W.D. (2002). Contextualized behavioral support in early intervention for children with autism and their families. *Journal of Autism and Developmental Disorders, 32*, 519–533.

Moes, D.R. Koegel, R.L., Schreibman, L., & Loos, L.M. (1992). Stress profiles for mothers and fathers of children with autism. *Psychological Reports, 71*, 1272–1274.

Murphy, M., Bolton, P.F., Pickles, A., Fombonne, E., Piven, J., & Rutter, M. (2000). Personality traits of the relatives of autistic probands. *Psychological Medicine, 30*, 1411–1424.

Narayan, S., Moyes, B., & Wolff, S. (1990). Family characteristics of autistic children: A further report. *Journal of Autism and Developmental Disorders, 20*, 523–535.

Netley, C., Lockyer, L., & Greenbaum, G.H.C. (1975). Parental characteristics in relation to diagnosis and neurological status in childhood psychosis. *British Journal of Psychiatry, 127*, 440–444.

O'Moore, M. (1968). Living with autism. *The Irish Journal of Psychology, 4*, 33–52.

Ornitz, E.M. & Ritvo, E.R. (1968). Perceptual inconstancy in the syndrome of early infant autism and its variants. *Archives of General Psychiatry, 18*, 76–98.

Piven, J. (1999). Genetic liability for autism: The behavioral expression in relatives. *International Review of Psychiatry, 11*, 299–308.

Piven, J., Chase, G.A., Landa, R., Wzorek, M., Gayle, J., Cloud, D. et al. (1991). Psychiatric disorders in the parents of autistic individuals. *Journal of the American Academy of Child & Adolescent Psychiatry, 30*, 471–478.

Piven, J. & Palmer, P. (1997). Cognitive deficits in parents from multiple-incidence autism families. *Journal of Child Psychology & Psychiatry & Allied Disciplines, 38*, 1011–1021.

Piven, J. & Palmer, P. (1999). Psychiatric disorder and the broad autism phenotype: Evidence from a family study of multiple-incidence autism families. *American Journal of Psychiatry, 156*, 557–563.

Piven, J., Palmer, P., Jacobi, D., Childress, D., & Arndt, S. (1997). Broader autism phenotype: Evidence from a family history study of multiple-incidence autism families. *American Journal of Psychiatry, 154*, 185–190.

Piven, J., Palmer, P., Landa, R., Santangelo, S., Jacobi, D., & Childress, D. (1997). Personality and language characteristics in parents from multiple-incidence autism families. *American Journal of Medical Genetics, 74*, 398–411.

Piven, J., Wzorek, M., Landa, R., Lainhart, J., Bolton, P., Chase, G.A. et al. (1994). Preliminary communication: Personality characteristics of the parents of autistic individuals. *Psychological Medicine, 24*, 783–795.

Plienis, A.J., Robbins, F.R., & Dunlap, G. (1988). Parent adjustment and family stress as factors in behavioral parent training for young autistic children. *Journal of the Multihandicapped Person, 1*, 31–52.

Pollack, R. (1997). *The Creation of Dr. B: A biography of Bruno Bettelheim.* New York: Simon and Schuster.

Rimland, B. (1964). *Infantile autism: The syndrome and its implications for a neural theory of behavior.* East Norwalk, CT: Appleton-Century-Crofts.

Ritvo, E.R., Cantwell, D., Johnson, E., Clements, M., Benbrook, F., Slagle, S. et al. (1971). Social class factors in autism. *Journal of Autism and Childhood Schizophrenia, 1*, 297–310.

Robbins, F.R., Dunlap, G., & Plienis, A. J. (1991). Family characteristics, family training, and the progress of young children with autism. *Journal of Early Intervention, 15*, 173–184.

Rodrigue, J.R., Morgan, S.B., & Geffken, G.R. (1990). Families of autistic children: Psychological functioning of mothers. *Journal of Clinical Child Psychology, 9*, 371–379.

Rodrigue, J.R., Morgan, S.B., & Geffken, G.R. (1992). Psychosocial adaptation of fathers of children with autism, Down syndrome, and normal development. *Journal of Autism and Developmental Disorders, 22*, 249–263.

Rutter, M. (1965). Influence of organic and emotional factors on the origins, nature and outcome of childhood psychosis. *Developmental Medicine and Child Neurology, 7*, 518–528.

Rutter, M. (1968). Concepts of autism: A review of research. *Journal of Child Psychology and Psychiatry & Allied Disciplines, 9*, 1–25.

Rutter, M. and Lockyer, L. (1967). A five to fifteen year follow-up study of infantile infantile psychosis: I Description of sample. *British Journal of Psychiatry, 113*, 169–1182.

Sanders, J.L. & Morgan, S.B. (1997). Family stress and adjustment as perceived by parents of children with autism or Down Syndrome: Implications for intervention. *Child & Family Behavior Therapy, 1997, 19*, 15–32.

Sauna, V.D. (1987). Infantile autism and parental socioeconomic status: A case of bimodal distribution. *Child Psychiatry and Human Development, 17*, 189–198.

Schopler, E. (1966). Visual versus tactual receptor preference in normal and schizophrenic children. *Journal of Abnormal Psychology, 71*, 108–114.

Schopler, E. (1995). *Parents' survival manual: A guide to crisis resolution in autism and related developmental disorders.* New York: Plenum Press.

Schopler, E. (1997). Implementation of TEACCH Philosophy. In D.J. Cohen & F.R. Volkmar (Eds.), *Handbook of autism and pervasive developmental disorders* (pp. 767–795). New York: John Wiley & Sons.

Schopler, E. (Ed.). (2000). International priorities for developing autism services via the TEACCH model [Special Issue]. *International Journal of Mental Health, 29(1)*.

Schopler, E., Andrews, C.E., & Strupp, K. (1979). Do autistic children come from upper-middle-class parents? *Journal of Autism and Developmental Disorders, 9*, 139–152.

Schopler, E., Mesibov, G.B., & Baker, A. (1982). Evaluation of treatment for autistic children and their parents. *Journal of the American Academy of Child Psychiatry, 21*, 262–267.

Schopler, E., Mesibov, G.B., Shigley, R.H., & Bashford, A. (1984). Helping autistic children through their parents: The TEACCH model. In E. Schopler & G.B. Mesibov (Eds.), *The effects of autism on the family* (pp. 65–81). New York: Plenum Press.

Schopler, E. & Reichler, R.J. (1971). Parents as cotherapists in the treatment of psychotic children. *Journal of Autism and Childhood Schizophrenia, 1*, 87–102.

Schreibman, L., Koegel, R.L., Mills, D.L., & Burke, J.C. (1984). Training parent-child interactions. E. Schopler & G.B Mesibov (Eds.), *The effects of autism on the family* (pp. 187–205). New York: Plenum Press.

Schreibman, L. (1997). Theoretical perspectives on behavioral intervention for individuals with autism. In D.J. Cohen & F.R. Volkmar (Eds.), *Handbook of autism and pervasive developmental disorders* (pp. 920–933). New York: John Wiley & Sons.

Sharpley, C.F., Bitsika, V., & Efremidis, B. (1997). Influence of gender, parental health, and perceived expertise of assistance upon stress, anxiety, and depression among parents of children with autism. *Journal of Intellectual & Developmental Disability, 22*, 19–28.

Shields, J. (2001). The NAS EarlyBird Programme: Partnership with parents in early intervention. *Autism, 5*, 49–56.

Short, A.B. (1984). Short-term treatment outcome using parents as co-therapists for their own autistic children. *Journal of Child Psychology & Psychiatry & Allied Disciplines, 25*, 443–458.

Sivberg, B. (2002). Family system and coping behaviors. *Autism, 6*, 397–409.

Smalley, S., McCracken, J., & Tanguay, P. (1995). Autism, affective disorders, and social phobia. *American Journal of Medical Genetics, 60*, 19–26.

Smith, T., Groen, A.D., & Wynn, J.W. (2000). Randomized trial of intensive early intervention for children with pervasive developmental disorder. *American Journal on Mental Retardation, 105*, 269–285.

Smith, T., Groen, A.D., & Wynn, J.W. (2001). "Randomized trial of intensive early intervention for children with pervasive developmental disorder." Errata. *American Journal on Mental Retardation, 106*, 208. Abstract retrieved November 12, 2002 from PsychINFO database.

Sofroroff, K. & Farbotko, M. (2002). The effectiveness of parent management training to increase self-efficacy in parents of children with Asperger syndrome. *Autism, 6*, 271–286.

Stahmer, A.C. & Gist, K. (2001). The effects of an accelerated parent education program on technique mastery and child outcome. *Journal of Positive Behavior Interventions, 3*, 75–82.

Steinhausen, H-C., Göbel, D., Breinlinger, M., & Wohlleben, B. (1986). A community survey of infantile autism. *Journal of the American Academy of Child Psychiatry, 25*, 186–189.

Stiebel, D. (1999). Promoting augmentative communication during daily routines. *Journal of Positive Behavior Interventions, 1*, 159–169.

Symon, J. B. (2001). Parent education for autism: Issues in providing services at a distance. *Journal of Positive Behavior Interventions, 3*, 160–174.

Treffert, D.A. (1970). Epidemiology of infantile autism. *Archives of General Psychiatry, 22*, 431–438.

Tsai, L., Stewart, M.A., Faust, M., & Shook, S. (1982). Social class distribution of fathers of children enrolled in the Iowa Autism Program. *Journal of Autism and Developmental Disorders, 12*, 211–221.

Tunali, B. & Power, T.G. (2002). Coping by redefinition: Cognitive appraisals in mothers of children with and without autism. *Journal of Autism and Developmental Disorders, 32*, 25–34.

Warren, F. (1984). The role of the national society in working with families. In E. Schopler & G.B. Mesibov (Eds.), *The effects of autism on the family* (pp. 99–115). New York: Plenum Press.

Weiss, M.J. (2002). Hardiness and social support as predictors of stress in mothers of typical children, children with autism, and children with mental retardation. *Autism, 6*, 115–130.

Whitaker, P. (2002). Supporting families of preschool children with autism: What parents want and what helps. *Autism, 6*, 411–426.

Wing, J.K. (1966). Diagnosis, epidemiology, aetiology. In J.K. Wing (Ed.). *Early childhood autism: Clinical, educational, and social aspects* (pp. 3–38). New York: Pergamon Press.

Wing, L. (1980). Childhood autism and social class: A question of selection? *British Journal of Psychiatry, 137*, 410–417.

Wolf, L.C., Noh, S., Fisman, S.N., & Speechley, M. (1989). Brief report: Psychological effects of parenting stress on parents of autistic children. *Journal of Autism and Developmental Disorders, 19*, 157–166.

CHAPTER 9

Providing Diagnostic Information to Parents

INTRODUCTION

When parents understand their child's developmental problems and special needs, they can obtain services, they can connect with other parents for support and mutual assistance, and they can form coalitions to advocate for more and better services and for research into treatment and prevention. However, initially learning about their child's significant developmental problems is very distressing for most parents. First hearing the words "autism" and "mental retardation" is one of their worst nightmares come true, with fear, pain, grief, disbelief, rage, and heartache flooding them as the professional talks. Although professionals in psychology, education, medicine, etc. chose their careers in order to help people, not to cause them distress, the very nature of telling parents that their child has a developmental disability involves inflicting extraordinary pain. So the process of explaining developmental test results to parents can be difficult for professionals as well as for parents (Abrams & Goodman, 1998; Lipton & Svarstad, 1977; Nissenbaum, Tollefson, & Reese, 2002).

But the problem exists whether it is named or not. The youngster still has significant needs, whether the parents understand them or not. Educational techniques, special therapies, and other interventions are available to make the person's future better, if only parents knew what was needed and how to get it. So for the sake of the child, the problem must be named and faced.

RESEARCH LITERATURE

The settings in which parents are told for the first time about their child's developmental disabilities are often called "interpretive sessions" or "informing interviews." The research literature related to these sessions is very small, while the clinical literature is somewhat more extensive (e.g., Doernberg, 1982; Miller, 1979; Morgan, 1984; Shea 1984, 1993).

Matheny and Vernick (1969) were among the first to question the prevailing professional view at that time that parents typically were so devastated by learning of their child's diagnosis of mental retardation that they distorted or rejected the information and needed at least short-term psychotherapy. In a paper titled "Parents of the Mentally Retarded Child: Emotionally Overwhelmed or Informationally Deprived?" Matheny and Vernick demonstrated a significant shift in parents' expectations about the child's future accomplishments (in the direction of more realistic expectations) following the receipt of information and answers to questions from pediatrician who had evaluated the child. These parents also followed the clinicians' recommendations to a very high degree.

The few studies involving direct analysis of the effects of different types of interpretive content have yielded similarly clear results. Svarstad and Lipton (1977) compared the audiotapes of 37 informing interviews at a multidisciplinary child development center with the written reports of the same children's evaluations. Based on this comparison, they derived scores for the frankness and completeness of the verbal information the professionals gave to parents. Comparing these results with the parents' understanding of their children's disabilities before and after the informing interviews, they found a significant relationship between the frankness and completeness of the information the professionals gave and higher parental acceptance of their children's mental retardation. However, they found that in almost half the sessions they studied, information was either vague, misleading, or omitted, which not surprisingly was associated with significantly lower levels of parental acceptance.

Cunnningham, Morgan, and McGucken (1984) compared parental satisfaction ratings before and after a model process for informing parents about their infants' Down Syndrome was introduced into a regional public health program. The elements of the model program were having the diagnosis given 1) in a private setting, 2) to both parents, 3) by a pediatrician, 4) with the baby present, 5) with time for questions, 6) with both general availability of the professionals and specific plans for additional contacts in the near future, and 7) with privacy for the parents after the diagnostic session. Before the model program, the researchers documented many typical criticisms of the informing process (that is, parents reported that they were told abruptly or unsympathetically; had limited information and limited opportunity to ask questions; were not told soon enough). The families who were informed as part of the model process had *no* criticisms about the process.

Brogan and Knussen (2003) analyzed parents' overall satisfaction with interpretive sessions in relation to their ratings of specific variables. They reported significant positive correlations between overall satisfaction and parents' views of the *quality of the information* (a summary of the amount of information they received, how technical it was, and their ability to understand and remember it) and with the *professional's manner* (a summary of whether the professional was sympathetic, approachable, direct as opposed to evasive, and a good communicator).

Another line of recent research has looked at interpretive sessions from the perspective of sociolingustic analysis (Abrams & Goodman, 1998; Bartolo, 2002; Gill & Maynard, 1995). These studies have found that there are certain characteristic patterns of informing parents of assessment results. These include asking parents for their perspectives then connecting the diagnostic information to elements of the parents' responses ("Perspective-Display series"), presenting information in small increments that enable parents to draw their own conclusions ("Incomplete Syllogism"), and using euphemisms and hedging (such as "slow," "delayed," "sort of," "I think").

Further, Abrams and Goodman (1998) used the term "negotiation" (p. 87) to describe some of the interactions between professionals and parents during interpretive sessions. By this they meant that professionals and parents reacted to each others' statements in ways that led to modifications, clarifications, or other changes in their original statements or positions. Specifically, they documented "negotiations" related to diagnostic labels and to degrees of optimism or pessimism regarding future functioning. They found that parents tended to ask questions about the diagnostic terms that often resulted in professionals' changing or qualifying the terms in some way (sometimes in the direction of reducing severity, sometimes in the direction of increasing clarity, because few of the professionals spontaneously used clear labels). The researchers characterized the professionals' reluctance to use clear labels as problematic, writing that "the professionals' habit of blurring diagnostic information invited parents to join in a struggle over the appropriate designation" (p. 91). They also found empirical evidence against the use of euphemisms and hedging instead of clear labels: in the final 10 minutes of interpretive sessions, parents who had not received the label of mental retardation asked significantly more questions, indicating higher levels of confusion. In terms of interactions related to prognosis, Abrams and Goodman found that professionals often made statements intended to balance very pessimistic *or* very optimistic expressions by parents. The researchers saw this type of "negotiation" as having beneficial aspects, writing that "the negotiation around pessimism/optimism serves two purposes: it presses the diagnosis and prognosis forward, while it keep parents at a level of tolerable comfort" (p. 96).

Researchers who have asked parents about their experiences in interpretive sessions have generally found several common themes. First, parents want clear information and direct answers (Midence & O'Neill, 1999; Quine & Pahl, 1987; Sloper & Turner, 1993). Second, parents are much more satisfied with the informing process when professionals are sympathetic and understanding of their feelings and reactions (Quine & Rutter, 1994). Third, parents want to know sooner rather than later, and want to know as much as possible (Quine & Pahl, 1986). Fourth, opportunities to ask questions and hear information repeated and re-explained are important (Quine & Pahl, 1986; Sloper & Turner, 1993).

Nissenbaum et al. (2002) interviewed a sample of parents and experienced professionals and developed the following recommendations: "1) become knowledgeable about autism; 2) establish a family-friendly setting; 3) understand the family's needs; 4) use good communication skills; 5) provide a list of resources and interventions; 6) provide follow-up; 7) discuss prognosis; 8) provide hope; 9) recognize that it is not unusual for professionals to react to giving the diagnosis of autism" such as feeling nervous, sad, self-doubting, and/or physiologically uncomfortable (p. 37).

In summary, the research and clinical literature suggests the importance of diagnostic information that is both direct and compassionate, that is both realistic and encouraging about the future, that is thorough, timely, and practical, and that provides a mechanism for asking questions and discussing issues. Although giving this information to parents can be distressing for professionals, it is fundamentally a benevolent act towards both the parents and the child.

TEACCH APPROACH TO SHARING DIAGNOSTIC INFORMATION WITH PARENTS

Overview

Interpretive practices within the TEACCH program are consistent with the literature reviewed above. Interpretive sessions are conducted by the regional centers' Clinical Directors, who are doctoral-level clinical psychologists skilled in both technical knowledge about autism spectrum disorders (ASD) and in compassionate conversations with families. Interpretive sessions almost always take place on the day of the child's evaluation and last as long as families need, which provides time for explanations, examples, questions, discussions, emotional reactions, etc. Diagnostic terms are clearly stated and explained, and parents are also later provided with the formal written report of their child's evaluation and individualized recommendations. TEACCH Centers also have handouts of practical articles and resources that can be given to parents, as well as books that can be loaned out.

General Goals and Techniques

Interpretive sessions for ASD and/or other developmental disabilities should be very different from a dispassionate information exchange among professionals. Parents have passionate feelings about their child, and these deserve to be acknowledged and respected. While one goal of the interpretive session should be to provide accurate, understandable information about the child, a second, equally important goal is to support parents emotionally as they hear and respond to this information. Parents' emotions *belong* in the interpretive session. (Techniques for eliciting and supporting emotional expression will be discussed below). A third goal of an interpretive session should be to provide concrete guidance about next steps, such as follow-up appointments, telephone numbers for therapists or agencies, names of books to read, useful websites, etc.

In order to achieve these goals, professionals should think through what they are going to say and how they are going to say it. This does not mean reading from a script; there must be genuine, personal dialogue among the participants. However, when professionals are aware of and thoughtful about the *process* of the discussion, its *setting and structure*, and the *content* they provide, they are most helpful to parents.

The Interpretive Process

The process of the interpretive session refers to the way information is presented. The essential theme for professionals to remember is to *balance honesty with compassion* (Shigley, personal communication, 1986). Together, these are powerful and beneficial to families; detached, they render the interpretive session either unkind or unhelpful.

Small acts and details in the interpretive process can make a difference in the quality of the session. In clinics with many staff members, it is advisable to begin the session by re-introducing all of the participants, since parents will have met many people during the course of the child's evaluation. Many professionals find it helpful to speak from a single page of notes (including the child's name and age, since professionals can be emotionally stressed and forgetful during the session too), diagnostic information, and recommendations, in order to be sure that all important points are included. *It is vital that professionals speak slowly.* The information being presented is both cognitively complex and emotionally charged. All parents, even highly educated ones, need time to process what is being said. It is possible to use complex sentences and advanced vocabulary with some families, but the professional's rate of speech should still be slower than it would be in a staff meeting or personal conversation. And certainly with many families, plain language must be used in place of professional jargon.

Professionals can set the tone of an honest yet compassionate discussion by responding to indications of feelings from parents. It is vital that the professionals watch parents' faces for indications of their feelings and concerns. For example, if parents become teary, it is very appropriate to make a comment like "this is very sad to think about" or "I know this is painful for you." If parents look as though they disagree with what is being said, the professional should take the initiative to say something like "Is this different from what you think?" or "Do you think we're wrong about this?" If parents appear confused by the information, a statement such as "I am not sure I am explaining this well – let me try again" can be helpful, as can encouraging the parents to ask questions about anything they would like to have explained more fully.

Occasionally parents strongly disagree with the diagnostic findings and labels, or are angry or defensive. It is not helpful to argue or debate the merits of the assessment in such situations. It is generally more useful to reflect and respect the parents' views, perhaps even indicating "I understand what you are saying and I hope you are right. However, in our experience ... (children with this pattern of development usually don't catch up; youngsters of this age with symptoms in the three areas that define autism spectrum disorders usually continue to have special needs into adulthood, etc.). We want to do everything that we can to help him achieve as much as possible."

A common reaction of some parents is to feel overwhelmed by the information. This often manifests itself as a blank or inattentive expression with limited eye contact. The best approach for professionals in this situation is to *stop talking*. The parent is obviously not processing what is being said at that point, and is caught up with internal thoughts and feelings. This is a very normal reaction to upsetting news or events. *Silence* at this point in the interpretive session is more supportive than anything else the professional can say, and is certainly more useful than continuing with a presentation of test results or recommendations. The professional can say something like "Let me stop for a minute so you can think about this" then simply sit in silence, looking neither embarrassed nor impatient, as the parent cries, or thinks, or copes with the waves of feelings that have been generated. After several minutes, if the parent has not resumed the conversation (which is rare), the professional can make general expressions of support and concern. Whatever seems to be the predominant feeling or thought can be named in a gentle inquiry ("Are you worried about what the future holds for him?" "I know this is so very sad for you." "Are you thinking about how to tell the rest of the family?" "You seem to be really angry that this is happening to your family."). Many professionals, particularly those with non-mental health backgrounds, are inexperienced and uncomfortable with parents' expressions of feelings. Others are uncertain how to handle withdrawn or unexpressive parents. In both situations, a combination of silence and gentle probing of feelings is much more helpful than going on with the presentation of interpretive content.

Ironically, while respect and empathy for parents' pain are vital to good interpretive discussions, the session need not be entirely serious and morose. The child with ASD and/or other developmental disability is first of all a child, and almost always brings pleasure, warmth, and laughter to the family at times. Not only is it important to make reference to his strengths, appealing qualities, and unique personality, it is also acceptable to use humor judiciously in the interpretive session, if it is natural to the situation and to the participants. Amusing anecdotes and warm acceptance of the youngster's endearing qualities contribute to an atmosphere in the session of shared appreciation of that child, which can contribute to the family's comfort.

Structural Variables

The setting of the interpretive session is important, and should not be left to chance. Settings such as waiting rooms, shared classrooms, or other public places should be avoided. Interpretives should be take place in a private setting, with adult-size chairs positioned so that all participants can comfortably see and hear each other. Family members should have the option of sitting near each other or not, because this may be a source of support or additional stress, depending on the particular family's dynamics. There should *always* be Kleenex easily available in the room. Parents frequently cry when told of their child's developmental disabilities; this is normal and should be supported and accepted as such. Other details can also make a difference in the parents' comfort: For example, the room should not be too cold or too hot, since extreme temperatures can add to the family's stress. Further, interpretive sessions are more comfortable and therapeutic when participants are not hungry and when they have had the opportunity to use the restroom before the session begins. Attention to such details can truly make a difference between a setting that is perceived as kind and caring, or unfeeling. While the content that will be discussed will likely be unpleasant, there is no reason that the setting and process cannot be made as comfortable as possible.

Parents who live together should both be present if at all possible. Otherwise, the parent who *is* present does not have the support of his or her partner, and then in addition has the responsibility of going home to explain complicated, distressing information to the other parent. Sometimes professionals must make advance plans or adjust their schedules to include both parents; while this is not always possible, it is generally the best practice in terms of family-centered care. In situations of family discord, some parents prefer not to have the other parent present, and this should be respected, while bearing in mind that state laws generally support the right of both parents to have equal access to information about their minor children, even when only one of them has custody. Separate interpretive sessions may need to be scheduled. What should be avoided is for professionals to exclude a parent on the basis of standard scheduling practices that may not be sensitive to a particular family's situation. Interpretive sessions should also be open to others whom the parents wish to have there, such as grandparents or workers from other agencies.

Interpretive sessions should not involve a large number of professionals, because this tends to interfere with including emotional topics and concerns in the discussion. Thus, for example, the practice in multi-disciplinary clinics of having four or more staff members present their findings during the same session is likely to overwhelm parents and move the focus from a supportive, holistic discussion of the child's needs to a technical, professionally-focused meeting. The staff to family ratio should generally not exceed 3:2 or 2:1. In TEACCH centers, the interpretive is usually conducted by the Clinical Director (a clinical psychologist) along with one or two other staff members who have spent much of the diagnostic day with the family.

Interpretive Content

Unless other factors, discussed below, suggest otherwise, an interpretive should typically include the *name, nature,* and *severity* of the child's disorder. In addition, the issues of *causes and future course* often need to be addressed. Specifically, whatever terms are standard and technically correct for the child's difficulties and will be used in written materials should be told to the parents. In addition, the meaning of these terms in simple terms should be explained. The severity of the disorder should be placed in perspective, ranging from a borderline or subtle manifestation to mild, moderate, or severe/significant/very serious. Although these latter words can be difficult to say as well as to hear, honesty and completeness are important standards for the professional to meet. The cause of the disorder may not be known, but parents generally wonder and worry about this, and professionals should be prepared to discuss what is known, what is not known, how to look for additional information about etiology if this is important to the parents, and what worries and fears about causality can be put to rest. Professionals should also be sensitive to parents' worries about the future of the child's development. To the extent that general projections about the future can be made (especially reassuring ones), professionals should consider including this information in their presentation, and should definitely respond to parents' questions in this regard.

Individualizing Interpretive Sessions

Although the information described above should be included in most interpretive sessions, the interaction of three additional factors determines how these sessions should be individualized for each family.

Family Concerns

First is the nature of the family's questions or concerns, since addressing these should take high priority in deciding the content and sequence of what will be covered in the interpretive session. It is therefore vital to explore these questions and concerns as part of the diagnostic process, so that plans can be made and resources identified in preparation for the interpretive session. For example, if the family is mainly concerned about a particular behavior, or a specific decision that must be made, or help in obtaining a particular service, then responding to these concerns must be included in the interpretive discussion, even if this means postponing the presentation of other material.

Family concerns are heavily influenced by the age of the child (for example, a preschool child with issues of toilet training, sleep problems, or temper tantrums vs. an adolescent with issues of sexuality, vocational training, or frustrations because of not having friends). The information presented should be relevant to current concerns, rather than a standardized set of facts and recommendations.

The interpretive should have a different focus depending on whether the primary question is diagnostic or treatment-focused. If the parents already strongly suspect the diagnosis of ASD and/or mental retardation or have sought this evaluation as a second opinion, then the details of testing and diagnostic reasoning are not as important as a response to that question then concrete recommendations. On the other hand, if the parents know little about ASD or mental retardation, then much more time must be spent explaining the nature of these disorders.

Another aspect of parents' concerns that should be considered in planning interpretive content is whether their focus is on home issues, school issues, or both. The most difficult situations for professionals are those in which questions or concerns involve the school/daycare/day program, but at the time of the conference limited information or contact with that program is available. It is difficult to make good recommendations for situations which are only poorly understood, and unwise to make recommendations to people who have not asked for them. Therefore, if professionals are to be helpful with situations related to school or other programs or agencies, follow-up contacts must be made.

Diagnosis

The second variable determining the content of an interpretive should be the nature of the child's developmental status and diagnosis. Interpretives have very different content and emotional tone depending on whether ASD and mental retardation are present, ruled out, or questionable.

Some individuals referred for evaluation of a possible ASD do not have the disorder. They may have other significant developmental or emotional concerns, but at least ASD can be ruled out. In these situations, the issue of ASD should generally be discussed first and dispensed with, before going on to cover other findings and recommendations. Doing this relieves parents' fears, and makes it more possible for them to participate with an easier spirit in the rest of the session.

When the diagnosis of ASD is being explained, a description of the three areas of symptomatology can be given, using examples from this individual's behavior during the evaluation or based on parent's descriptions from home. For example, "In the area of *communication*, we could see that Jeff repeats a lot of things that are said to him, but has a harder time following verbal directions, particularly unfamiliar directions such as 'stand up and jump.' He also had a hard time using his language to ask for things directly, and he wasn't really able to answer questions or engage in a conversation. We could also see, and you told us, that he has *social* problems: He wasn't very interested in getting attention from the people who were working with him today, and you told us that he doesn't try to seek out other children in your neighborhood or at school. Finally, we could see that Jeff did have some *unusual play interests and behaviors*. He liked to tear up paper and watch it fall, just the way you said he does at home, he wasn't interested in many of the toys in the room except for the ones that he could spin, and at times he held his hands in unusual ways and looked at them. These three areas, communication, social skills and interests, and unusual ways of playing, are all symptoms of autism. So we are saying that the diagnosis of autism does apply to Jeff."

Whether or not the individual has ASD, mental retardation may be identified during the evaluation. This is often the more painful diagnosis for parents to hear. As a result, perhaps, there is a philosophical movement in some parts of the developmental disabilities community against diagnosing or talking about mental retardation with parents. However, mental retardation exists, it can be identified at some point in development, and if a youngster has mental retardation the parents have a right to know, so professionals have an obligation to tell them.

In certain circumstances it may be appropriate for professionals to refrain from using the term "mental retardation." These circumstances would include 1) a very young child (under age three years) with significant developmental scatter, such that a summary score in the range of mental retardation does not reflect indications of higher potential; 2) factors in the child's history that may make current developmental status of questionable use in predicting future development (for example, prolonged hospitalization or environmental deprivation, or early learning in a different language environment; 3) psychologically fragile parents; 4) parents with mental retardation themselves, who may not obtain any useful information from use of the term; and 5) other clinical or social factors carefully considered by the professional before making a decision not to mention mental retardation for the time being.

Two other possible reasons for not talking about mental retardation are not appropriate: 1) the professionals' discomfort with the parents' feelings of grief or anger, and 2) capitulation to the current trend that 'if we don't give the problem a name it won't exist' or 'if we change its name, we change its nature or severity.' As discussed earlier, parents' feelings of grief and fear are normal responses to the devastating news of a serious developmental disability. These feelings should be anticipated and accepted, not avoided. Although terms such as 'developmental delay' and 'pervasive developmental disorder' may at times be the most appropriate labels for young children or those with atypical symptomatology, those terms are too often used as euphemisms for mental retardation and autism. As discussed above, if the problem exists, to the extent that parents are left uninformed about it, they are less able to meet the youngster's needs.

Family Factors

Family members' intellectual and educational levels should also influence the content of the interpretive session. Both the kind of information presented and the amount should be individualized according to these factors. The lower the intelligence or education (these are not always correlated) the less information should be presented initially. Naturally, questions should be encouraged and answered, so if the professional has misjudged the family's intellectual level or knowledge, there is a mechanism for readjusting the type and amount of content.

Anther family factor to consider is the family members' psychological status. The shakier it is, the less distressing news professionals should present, while making arrangements for additional supports to be added to the system. Examples are parents with untreated bipolar disorder or depression, parents with a history of violence, or parents with significant substance abuse problems. Decisions about how and what to tell these parents should be carefully thought through *before* beginning the interpretive session.

SUMMARY

Consistent with the research literature on family preferences and effective practices, the TEACCH program values providing parents with honest, complete, and practical information about their child in an empathic, sensitive manner. This lays the foundation both for parents and professionals to work in partnership and also for parents to make the most informed plans and decisions for their youngsters.

REFERENCES

Abrams, E.Z. & Goodman, J.F. (1998). Diagnosing developmental problems in children: Parents and professionals negotiate bad news. *Journal of Pediatric Psychology, 23*, 87–98.

Bartolo, P.A. (2002). Communicating a diagnosis of developmental disability to parents: Multiprofessional negotiations frameworks. *Child: Care, Health & Development, 28*, 65–71.

Brogan, C.A. & Knussen, C. (2003). The disclosure of a diagnosis of an autistic spectrum disorder: Determinants of satisfaction in a sample of Scottish parents. *Autism, 7*, 31–46.

Cunningham, C.C., Morgan, P.A., & McGucken, R.B. (1984). Down's syndrome: Is dissatisfaction with disclosure of diagnosis inevitable? *Developmental Medicine and Child Neurology, 26*, 33–39.

Doernberg, N. (1982). Issues in communication between pediatricians and parents of young mentally retarded children. *Pediatric Annals, 11*, 438–444.

Gill, V.T. & Maynard, D.W. (1995). On "labeling" in actual interaction: Delivering and receiving diagnoses of developmental disabilities. *Social Problems, 42*, 11–37.

Lipton, H.L. & Svarstad, B. (1977). Sources of variation in clinicians' communication to parents about mental retardation. *American Journal of Mental Deficiency, 82*, 155–161.

Matheny, A.P. & Vernick, J. (1969). Parents of the mentally retarded child: Emotionally overwhelmed or informationally deprived? *The Journal of Pediatrics, 74*, 953–959.

Midence, K. & O'Neill, M. (1999). The experience of parents in the diagnosis of autism. *Autism, 3*, 273–285.

Miller, N.B. (1979). Parents of children with neurological disorders: Concerns and counseling. *Journal of Pediatric Psychology, 4*, 297–306.

Morgan, S.B. (1984). Helping parents understand the diagnosis of autism. *Developmental and Behavioral Pediatrics, 5*, 78–85.

Nissenbaum, M.S., Tollefson, N., & Reese, R.M. (2002). The interpretive conference: Sharing a diagnosis of autism with families. *Focus on Autism and Other Developmental Disabilities, 17*, 30–43.

Quine, L. & Pahl, J. (1986). First diagnosis of severe mental handicap: Characteristics of unsatisfactory encounters between doctors and parents. *Social Science and Medicine, 22*, 53–62.

Quine, L. & Pahl, J. (1987). First diagnosis of severe handicap: A study of parental reactions. *Developmental Medicine and Child Neurology, 29*, 232–242.

Quine, L. & Rutter, D.R. (1994). First diagnosis of severe mental and physical disability: A study of doctor-parent communication. *Journal of Child Psychology and Psychiatry, 35*, 1273–1287.

Shea, V. (1984). Explaining mental retardation and autism to parents. In E. Schopler & G.B. Mesibov (Eds.), *The effects of autism on the family* (pp. 265–288). New York: Plenum Press.

Shea, V. (1993). Interpreting results to parents of preschool children. In E. Schopler, M.E. Van Bourgondien, & M. Bristol (Eds.), *Preschool issues in autism* (pp. 185–198). New York: Plenum Press.

Sloper, P. & Turner, S. (1993). Determinants of parental satisfaction with disclosure of disability. *Developmental Medicine and Child Neurology, 35*, 816–825.

Svarstad, B.L. & Lipton, H.L. (1997). Informing parents about mental retardation: A study of professional communication and parent acceptance. *Social Science and Medicine, 11*, 645–651.

CHAPTER 10

Preschool Issues

INTRODUCTION

The preschool years provide a critical foundation for later learning and development (Guralnick, 1998; Ramey & Ramey, 1998) and they may be particularly important for children with autism spectrum disorders (ASD; Fenske, Zalenski, Krantz, & McClannahan, 1985; Harris & Handelman, 2001). Limited skills and rigid, repetitive behaviors have the potential to interfere greatly with children's learning and participation in family life and in their communities. Early intervention services are a vital part of the often lifelong attempt to decrease the functional impact of ASD. Several recent advances in our understanding of early childhood and autism highlight the considerable significance of services for young children with ASD.

First, the diagnosis of an autism spectrum disorder can be reliably made at increasingly younger ages. Researchers have been able to identify behavioral deficits that distinguish children with autism in the first year of life (Baranek, 1999; Maestro et al., 2002; Osterling, Dawson, & Munson, 2002; Werner, Dawson, Osterling, & Dinno, 2000). These results were based on fine-grained analyses of videotaped behavior, not real-time clinical observation, but the behavioral deficit of 'lack of response to name' at age one year is so common that it may be observable during typical clinical interactions such as doctor visits (Rogers, 2001). It should be noted, however, that there is also increasing empirical support for the existence of 'late onset' autism, which does not become evident until after the first year of life (Osterling et al., 2002).

With regard to the toddler years, advances in early screening and diagnostic practices clearly allow clinicians to identify children with autism more accurately than in the past (Lord & Risi, 2000). Rogers (2001) summarized the research literature as follows: "Clinicians looking for autism need to be alert for toddlers who demonstrate relatively typical play for developmental level with toddler-level cause and effect or sensorimotor toys but little or no pretend play, relatively severe developmental delays according to infant development tests, a history of normal or near normal motor development, and lack of expected language, social, and gestural development for nonverbal developmental level" (p. 17).

Similarly, a multidisciplinary consensus panel of representatives from nine professional organizations (e.g., American Academy of Child and Adolescent Psychiatry, American Academy of Neurology, American Academy of Pediatrics, American Psychological Association), the National Institutes of Health, and four parent organizations completed an extensive literature review and developed guidelines for screening for and diagnosing ASD (Filipek et al., 1999). These guidelines included the following "absolute indications for immediate further evaluation: 1) no babbling by 12 months; 2) no gesturing (pointing, waving bye-bye, etc. by 12 months); 3) no single words by 16 months; 4) no 2-word spontaneous *(not just echolalic)* phrases by 24 months; 5) ANY loss of ANY language or social skills at ANY age" (p. 452); the guidelines also outline other observations in the areas of communication, social skills, and atypical behaviors that should be considered "red flags for autism" (p. 452).

A second recent development that highlights the importance of developing early childhood services is the growing number of young children identified with an ASD. Recent surveys suggest that the prevalence rate for ASD may be as high as approximately 60 per 10,000 (Baird et al., 2000; Bertrand et al., 2001; Chakrabarti & Fombonne, 2001). Fombonne (2003) noted that, based on this estimate, in the United States there are approximately 114,000 children under five years of age with an ASD.

Third, research has indicated the vital importance of early experiences in shaping language (Chandler, Christie, Newson, & Prevezer; Goldstein, 2002; Kaiser & Gray, 1993), social skills (Hwang & Hughes, 2000; McConnell, 2002; Mundy & Crowson, 1997; Strain & Hoyson, 2000), and brain development (Bristol et al., 1996; Fischer & Rose, 1994).

Although it is clear that the symptoms that comprise autism are the result of factors that influence the developing brain, the precise links between pathophysiology and behavior are not well understood. Currently, interventions that emphasize skill acquisition across various domains (academic, self-help, socialization, play, and communication) are the primary focus of treatment for children with ASD (National Research Council, 2001).

LEGAL FOUNDATIONS FOR PRESCHOOL SERVICES

In 1986, the US Congress passed Public Law 99-457 (Education of Handicapped Children Act) which provided incentives for states to extend to 3–5 year old children with disabilities the same access to a free, appropriate public education (FAPE) that since 1975 had been a mandated program for 6–18 year old students. This law also established the voluntary (for states) Program for Infants and Toddlers with Disabilities (from birth through 2 years). Individual states had some leeway to select specific services provided, the date they were phased in, the definition of populations eligible for the services, the administrative organization of services, and the level of state funding, but by 1992–93 all states and the District of Columbia provided FAPE to 3–5 year old children with disabilities (including autism) and since 1994 all states have provided early intervention (birth through 2 years) services as well (Trohanis, 2002).

SERVICE PROVISION MODELS

The final regulations of the most recent (1997) amendment of the Federal special education law included the provision for children through 2 years of age that "to the maximum extent appropriate to the needs of the child, early intervention services must be provided in natural environments, including the home and community settings in which children without disabilities participate" (http://www.ideapractices.org/law/index.php). For many children, particularly those from birth through age 2 years, this means receiving publicly-funded services at home (or in a babysitter's home) from an itinerant early intervention specialist. Other infants and toddlers are served through periodic visits from an early intervention specialist to the child's placement in a typical child care facility, such as a day care center or local preschool program.

Services in natural environments may continue after 3 years of age (and the relevant section of federal regulations requires that "to the maximum extent appropriate, children with disabilities . . . are educated with children who are non-disabled"; http://www.ideapractices.org/law/index.php) but in addition to providing services in other settings, many states, through their local school districts, provide preschool special education classrooms beginning at age 3 years.

In local public school classrooms, particularly in small, poor, or rural school districts, there are usually not enough children with ASD or sufficient resources to provide autism-specific preschool classrooms. Thus, many preschoolers with ASD attend non-categorical preschool special education classrooms that also serve children with mental retardation, sensory impairments, motor impairments, speech/language disorders, and severe behavior problems.

However, many educators, clinicians, and researchers have recognized that the unique learning styles and characteristics of children with ASD necessitate specialized strategies and programs. Attempts to employ typical early childhood teaching approaches are often frustrated by the different learning styles of young children with ASD, and generic early intervention or special education often does not effectively address the scattered skills and atypical behaviors of children with autism. Several university-affiliated autism programs have developed specialized programs for preschool children with ASD, including Rutgers University, the University of California at Los Angeles (UCLA), the State University of New York at Binghamton, the University of Colorado in Denver, Emory University, and the University of North Carolina—Chapel Hill. Descriptions of these and other specialized programs are contained in Handelman and Harris's book "Preschool Education Programs for Children with Autism" (2001).

CONTROVERSIES AND CONSENSUS

The topic of preschool services for ASD is quite contentious, both in the psychological and educational literature and in the courts. Various researchers and scholars have published critiques—and rebuttals—about each other's work (e.g., Gresham & McMillan 1997a, 1997b; Jordan, Jones, and Murray, 1998; Lovaas, 2002; Shea, in press; Smith & Lovaas, 1997) and there have been many due process hearings and court cases related to disagreements between parents and school systems about appropriate educational services (National Research Council, 2001).

However, although different theoretical approaches to ASD and early intervention have resulted in differences among techniques and programs, two trends leading toward reconciliation or blending of approaches are evident. First, various experts have cautioned against dogmatic adherence to one instructional strategy, and have supported the importance of matching the specific learning styles and characteristics of individual children and their families to treatment approaches and techniques, in order to produce optimal results. For example, a consensus panel of the National Institutes of Health (Bristol et al., 1996) concluded that "treatments that are dramatically effective for one person with autism may be ineffective or even contraindicated for others" (p. 149). Heflin and Simpson (1998), in an article titled 'Interventions for Children and Youth with Autism: Prudent Choices in a World of Exaggerated Claims and Empty Promises' wrote that "the most effective programs for students with autism are those that incorporate a variety of best practices" (p. 207). Similarly, a recent workshop given in various locations nationally stressed the importance of an eclectic approach as a "component of a defensible program" for students with autism (Genaux and Maloney-Baird; videotape available from www.lrpdartnell.com). Further, Smith and Antolovich (2000) found that on average, parents in their sample (N = 121) had arranged for their children to have an average of 7 (range 0–15) interventions in addition to applied behavior analytic treatment.

Second, several recent literature reviews of autism-specific preschool programs have identified many commonalities among effective programs. For example, Dawson and Osterling (1997) reviewed eight well-known service models for preschool children with ASD, specifically the Douglass Developmental Disabilities Center, the Health Sciences Center Program at the University of Colorado in Denver, the LEAP program (Learning Experiences . . . An Alternative Program for Preschoolers and Parents), the May Institute, the Princeton Child Development Institute, the Walden Preschool at Emory University, the Young Autism Project at UCLA, and the TEACCH program at the University of North Carolina – Chapel Hill. The authors concluded that "all of the programs were quite effective in fostering positive school placement, significant developmental gains, or both for a substantial percentage of their students" (p. 314). They identified six factors they described as "basic shared beliefs and methods" that characterized the eight programs, "despite...different philosophical backgrounds and approaches" (p. 308). These factors were 1) the skills taught (specifically, paying attention to the environment, imitation, understanding and use of language, play with toys, and social interaction skills); 2) intensive teaching followed by systematic generalization; 3) predictability and routines; 4) behavior management that emphasized understanding the antecedents and functions of behavior; 5) programming with a goal of eventual independence; and 6) family involvement.

Rogers (1998) analyzed three of the same preschool service models (Colorado-Denver; UCLA, and TEACCH) from the perspective of their approaches to the neuropsychological differences that characterize ASD. She indicated that all three programs, in different ways, addressed these neuropsychological difficulties with 1) social interaction skills (referred to as "intersubjectivity"; p. 106); 2) imitation; 3) executive function; 4) emotion; 5) sensory and arousal issues; and 6) general rate of learning and development. Further, she wrote that "the importance of structured, systematized teaching using principles of learning theory, including breaking down tasks into small steps, teaching steps individually, and use of reinforcement for correct performance is recognized and practice by all of these models, though the surface language may differ" (p. 110).

Similarly, Hurth, Shaw, Izeman, Whaley, and Rogers (1999) described the results of a multi-stage consensus-building process with a group of experts from more than 20 programs for young children with autism. This process yielded agreement on six aspects of effective educational practice, and three additional elements that some, but not all of the experts agreed with. Principles yielding broad agreement were that 1) intervention should begin as early as possible in the child's life; 2) services should be individualized for children and families; 3) educational content should be planned and systematic; 4) educational content should reflect the particular characteristics and difficulties of ASD; 5) children should be engaged in learning activities for a large percentage of their time; and 6) families should be involved and supported in multiple ways. Additional topics on which there was agreement among some programs were 1) physical structure and a structured sequence of activities; 2) developmentally and culturally appropriate practices; 3) interventions in natural settings and with typically-developing peers.

Most recently, a panel of experts convened by the National Research Council (2001) again noted multiple similarities among 10 well-known comprehensive programs for young children with ASD, including many of those previously cited, and the Developmental Intervention Model at the George Washington University, the Individualized Support Program at the University of South Florida at Tampa, and the Pivotal Response Model at the University of California at Santa Barbara. Many of the common elements identified by other reviews were confirmed; additional common elements described in this report were 1) staff with extensive, specific training in autism; 2) ongoing assessment of students' progress; and 3) systematic programming for generalization of skills and transitions to the next educational environment. The panel rightly noted that of greater significance than philosophical or procedural difference *among* model programs, "the national challenge is to close the gap between the quality of model programs and the reality of most publicly funded early educational programs" (p. 140).

SUMMARY

In summary, there is evidence that ASD can be identified in very young children, and educational services are expanding to meet the needs of this growing population. Although professional and legal disputes continue among some proponents of particular programs, there is also growing awareness of the common elements in various well-known programs and of the importance of an eclectic combination of autism-specific educational techniques.

THE TEACCH APPROACH TO
PRESCHOOL EDUCATION

The TEACCH approach to educating students of any age is not a standard sequence of lesson plans and or standardized set of materials. Rather, it is a multifaceted approach to understanding individuals with ASD and providing them with the individualized supports they need in order to learn skills and develop as much independence as possible. Many of the techniques developed in other autism programs are not only compatible with, but are frequently integrated into TEACCH's work with students of all ages; these include traditional behavioral techniques (such as prompting, shaping, reinforcement, and response cost procedures) neo-behavioral approaches (such as incidental teaching and functional behavioral analysis) and developmentally appropriate practices.

As described earlier, early intervention and preschool special education programs in the United States are the legal and financial responsibility of state governments, provided through local school districts and other administrative units. However, at various times TEACCH has designed and operated one or more demonstration preschool classrooms. Described below is an example of what one TEACCH preschool looked like.

A STRUCTURED TEACHING
PRESCHOOL CLASSROOM

General Characteristics

The preschool classroom served five students, ages 3–5 years, all of whom had autism spectrum diagnoses, with varying degrees of developmental delay and severity of ASD. A lead teacher and assistant teacher staffed the class-room. Students attended preschool four hours per day, five days per week, and the preschool followed a traditional North Carolina school year calendar (early August—late May). The school day was composed of both highly structured and less structured activities using developmentally appropriate materials. Daily activities included direct one-to-one instruction, independent work sessions, small group activities, structured play, free play, gross motor activities, snack, and lunch. Some students also participated in small and large group activities with non-autistic peers and had speech/language, occupational, and/or physical therapies.

The classroom day was divided into 15-minute blocks of time or periods. Most frequently, students spent periods participating in structured learning ac-tivities with short breaks in the free play area between periods. Periods were divided differently for different students based on factors such as the student's ability to sustain attention, level of activity, and motivation. For example one student participated in two short one-to-one teaching sessions during a single period, while another student participated in a regular education classroom activity spanning two periods. The number of periods each student spent in various activities varied from student to student; one student had 4–6 daily one-to-one teaching sessions, while another child had one direct instruction session and participated in 2–3 small group activities. The classroom schedule was posted so that the teacher and assistant could clearly see which child was scheduled for which activity and which adult was responsible for each child's learning during each period.

Curriculum

The Preschool Curriculum Guide (see below) was individualized for each student based on formal and information evaluations at the beginning of the school year, and was adjusted to meet the changing needs of each student based on ongoing assessment throughout the school year. A battery of tests was administered to each student at the beginning of the school year. For-mal testing included the Psychoeducational Profile-Revised (PEP-R), Vineland Adaptive Behavior Scales-Parent Interview, and a measure of cognitive function-ing that varied from student to student. The assessment process also included speech/language and occupational and physical therapy evaluations when ap-propriate. The teacher used the information gathered through the assessment process to determine levels of functioning across developmental domains for the purpose of tailoring the curriculum to each student's strengths, interests, needs, and learning style.

The Curriculum Guide, which had been previously developed to assist the teacher in selecting and documenting teaching objectives, included eight func-tion areas: imitation; socialization and play with toys; language and commu-nication; readiness; adaptive behaviors; fine motor/eye-hand integration, gross motor, and self-help/daily living skills. Each function area delineated a series of skills that typically developing preschool aged children should know or be learning, and also included some higher-level skills that tapped the unique strengths and interests of some preschoolers with ASD. The teacher in the preschool classroom used the Curriculum Guide along with her general knowledge of child development, specific knowledge about each individual student, and parental input to develop the most appropriate curriculum for each student. She also ensured that each student's curriculum was broad, encompassing skills represented by all eight function areas.

Structured Teaching Strategies

TEACCH's Structured Teaching strategies (see Chapter 4, Structured Teaching) provided the foundation for learning in the preschool classroom. The classroom environment was highly physically structured. (Physical structure refers to the arrangement and organization of space and materials to create clearly defined learning areas.) Although typical preschoolers are generally able to segment their environments conceptually by understanding what materials "go together" (e.g. dolls, table, dishes, dress up clothes conceptually go together to create a "home living" center) the preschooler with ASD is more likely to focus on disconnected visual and physical details of the learning environment. In the TEACCH classroom, the teacher used naturally occurring boundaries such as walls and carpets, along with dividers and furniture, to create concrete and visually defined learning areas. The physical structure enabled the students to learn that certain activities were associated with specific clearly defined areas, and helped them learn the unique expectations for each area. For example, the student learned that the 1-to-1 area was where he went to work with the teacher and that the expectation was that the teacher would present new activities and provide directions and support, whereas the independent work area was where he went to work alone, completing activities that he had learned without receiving teacher direction or support.

Each student had an individualized daily schedule that visually and concretely helped him predict the sequence of activities that he would participate in each day. Schedules were individualized for each student in terms of what kind of visual cue was used to indicate activities or areas (objects, pictures, written words, or some combination of these), the length of the schedule (one at a time, sequence representing part of the day, sequence representing all of the day), and how the student interacted with his schedule to see that he was making progress in completing the activities on the schedule (took an object/picture from the schedule and carried it to the activity, turned over a picture or crossed off a written item before going to the activity). The schedule was used to ease transition times, build flexibility, increase understanding about expectations, help students learn to wait and anticipate, and help them to become increasingly independent.

Students were taught to complete individual activities by following their work/activity system. As described in Chapter 4, Structured Teaching, the work/activity system is an organizational strategy that visually and concretely answers four questions: What work (or activities) will I do? How much work will I do? How will I know that I am making progress toward being finished? and What happens next? The answers to these questions were provided in different ways for different students based on their learning style, strengths, and needs.

At the most basic level, activities to be done and a cue representing what the student would do when his activities were complete were placed on a surface to the student's left. The student was taught to take an activity from his left, complete it on the work area in front of him, and then to place it on a surface or in a container to his right. This procedure was to be repeated until all activities were complete. Thus, the activities were clearly organized so that the student could easily see *what* and *how much* work, could see that he was *finished* when the activities were gone from his left and placed on his right, and could see *what was next* because he had a symbol (or concrete material) on the table to his left that showed him. More developmentally advanced students instead used a matching or written work/activity system, which provided identical information to the student, but through the use of pictures or words.

The work/activity system was taught during direct one-to-one instruction sessions with a teacher, using any and all instructional techniques that the student understood, including traditional behavioral techniques of modeling, physical and verbal prompts that were eventually faded, reinforcement of successive approximations, and backward chaining. (Note that for many individuals with ASD, *finishing* activities appears to be a particularly powerful *positive* reinforcer.) Once the system was mastered in the one-to-one instruction setting, it was practiced in independent work sessions, then eventually incorporated into many of the activities that made up the student's day. For example, group activities, self-help tasks, and skill development activities could all be structured using elements of each student's work/activity system to help him understand 'what, how much, when finished, and what next.'

In addition, many of the developmentally typical learning activities used in the preschool classroom were structured in ways that were particularly engaging to young children with autism. For example, verbal instructions were accompanied or replaced by visual instructions to build on the relative visual strength of the majority of the preschool students. Language-based activities also had a visual or manipulative component (something to hold, look at, shake, touch, pass to someone, feel, etc.) to ensure that the students were actively engaged in the learning activity. Many activities also incorporated other skills, such as sorting and matching, that preschool children with ASD tend to be intrinsically motivated to attempt and complete. For example, when working on a language activity of identifying objects that belong to different categories, the teacher might have real objects or pictures of objects for the students to match or sort (e.g., put toys in the toy chest and animals in the toy farm).

In general, the specialized nature of the classroom had more to do with *how* skills were taught than with *what* skills and activities comprised the program. Visually structuring activities built on the strengths and interests of young students with ASD and supported engagement in learning typical preschool skills.

In addition to being a setting with visual and physical structure, sched-ules, and individualized programs, the preschool classroom was also a place for fun, laughter, warmth, social engagement, and incidental teaching. In particu-lar, time in the free play area was the setting where teachers observed students' preferences, followed their lead in playing with materials and interacting so-cially, engaged in imitation games, expanded on students' play, and used verbal labels for meaningful objects and actions. Snack time and lunch were also im-portant times for supporting communication development, both receptive and expressive.

Parental Participation

Parental participation was highly valued and sought in the preschool class-room. Parents served as collaborators with the teaching staff from the very begin-ning of their child's participation in the program. Parents participated in a semi-structured interview to complete the Vineland Adaptive Behavior Scales and provided the teaching staff with specific expertise about how autism affected their child. The teaching staff communicated daily with each family through the use of communication notebooks and/or direct contact during drop-off and pick-up times. This helped ensure continuity between environments and pro-moted flexible adjustments in programming based on observations of students' progress over time. Parents were invited to volunteer in the preschool classroom and on class outings. They were also invited to attend special programs such as open-house, holiday parties, and extra curricular events such as dance recitals.

Least Restrictive Environment

The preschool program was housed in a community facility that also housed a traditional preschool program for typically developing children. Students from the TEACCH classroom were integrated with the traditional preschool program peers in various ways depending on the specific learning style and needs of each student with ASD; specific considerations included their level of social comfort, their ability to manage stimulation, and their ability to imitate adults and peers. Some students spent the first hour of the day in a traditional preschool classroom participating in circle activities and centers, and some participated in a large group activity such as music, dance, or stories. Some of the students with ASD participated with non-autistic peers during specific therapies or for small group activities within the autism classroom, utilizing a 'reverse mainstreaming' model. Other students participated with non-autistic peers during gross motor activities such as outdoor recess or gym time. Overall, students with ASD were mainstreamed in ways that they could be successful—during those activities of the day that incorporated their strengths and interests. Most frequently the specific skills that they needed in order to be successful were taught within the Structured Teaching preschool class using the types of visual supports described previously, and then those supports (schedules, specific visual instructions, work/activity system) were incorporated into the more natural environments to support successful integration.

Evaluating Progress

Progress was measured in several ways in the preschool program. Progress on specific skills was documented on a daily basis and shared in written form with parents on at least a bi-weekly basis. Skills were not considered mastered until the student demonstrated mastery in multiple settings and with multiple people. For example, "sorting objects" would not be considered mastered until the student could sort many different kinds of objects into several different kinds of containers, during direct instruction, independent work, and small group sessions, and with the teacher and the teaching assistant. All students also had Individual Education Plans that were reviewed at least quarterly and updated yearly.

Pre- and post-preschool measures were obtained for students during a two-year period. For 12 of 13 children, age equivalents from the PEP-R (Psychoed-ucational Profile—Revised; Schopler, Reichler, Bashford, Lansing, and Marcus, 1990) were available from the period just prior to their entry into the preschool, and from May of that preschool year. Since children entered at different times of the school year, the lengths of the pre- and post-intervention period differed (range 5–9 months). All of the children made progress during the intervention period, and 8 of the 12 made more than one month's progress for every month that they were in the preschool. The ratio of 'overall PEP-R age equivalent months of progress' vs. 'months of time in the preschool' for the whole group (N = 12) was 1.49 (range .22 to 3.67; see Table 1). PEP-R scores were not

Table 10.1 Comparison of Progress and Time in Program

Student	Column A: Months of Progress, overall PEP-R age equivalent	Column B: Months in TEACCH Preschool	Ratio of Progress to Time in Program (Column A/Column B)
1	11.5	7	1.64
2	13	6	2.17
3	22	6	3.67
4	14	8	1.75
5	10.5	8	1.31
6	14.5	8	1.75
7	15	9	1.67
8	2	9	.22
9	7.5	9	.83
10	9	5	1.80
11	6.5	9	.72
12	4	9	.44

available for the 13th child, but he showed increases in standard scores on the Peabody Picture Vocabulary Test (from 'below 40' to 64), the Expressive One Word Picture Vocabulary Test (from 67 to 80), and the Leiter (from 83 to 95).

CONCLUDING COMMENTS

TEACCH provides services to individuals with autism of all ages, and it is not possible or appropriate to argue that one age group is more deserving than another. Nevertheless, the significance of early intervention/preschool services to young children with ASD cannot be overstated. There is increasing recognition of the shared elements of effective specialized programs for this population, and the flexible and multi-faceted nature of the TEACCH program incorporates virtually all of these important elements. The challenge now is to expand the availability of effective autism-specific interventions to all young children, and to focus public policies, personnel preparation, and research in support of this goal (National Research Council, 2001).

REFERENCES

Baird, G., Charman, T., Baron-Cohen, S., Cox, A, Swettenham, J., Wheelwright, S. et al. (2000). A screening instrument for autism at 18 months of age: A 6 year follow-up study. *Journal of the American Academy of Child and Adolescent Psychiatry, 3*, 694–702.

Baranek, G. (1999). Autism during infancy: A retrospective video analysis of sensory-motor and social behaviors at 9–12 months of age. *Journal of Autism and Developmental Disorders, 29*, 213–224.

Bertrand, J., Mars, A., Boyle, C., Bove, F., Yeargin-Allsopp, M., & Decoufle, P. (2001). Prevalence of autism in a United States population: The Brick Township, New Jersey, investigation. *Pediatrics, 108*, 1155–1161.

Bristol, M.M., Cohen, D.J., Costello, E.J., Denckla, M., Eckberg, T.J., Kallen, R. et al. (1996). State of the science in autism: Report to the National Institutes of Health. *Journal of Autism and Developmental Disorders, 26*, 121–154.

Chakrabarti, S. & Fombonne, E. (2001). Pervasive developmental disorders in preschool children. *Journal of the American Medical Association, 285*, 3093–3099.

Chandler, S., Christie, P., Newson, E., & Prevezer, W. (2002). Developing a diagnostic and intervention package for 2- to 3-year-olds with autism: Outcomes of the Frameworks for Communication approach. *Autism, 6*, 47–69.

Dawson, G. & Osterling, J. (1997). Early intervention in autism. In M. J. Guralnick (Ed.), *The effectiveness of early intervention* (pp. 307–326). Baltimore: Paul H. Brookes.

Fenske, E.C., Zalenski, S., Krantz, P.J., & McClannahan, L.E. (1985). Age at intervention and treatment outcome autistic children in a comprehensive intervention program. *Analysis and Intervention in Developmental Disabilities, 5*, 48–58.

Filipek, P.A., Accardo, P.J., Baranek, G.T., Cook, E.H., Dawson, G., Gordon, B. et al. (1999). The screening and diagnosis of autistic spectrum disorders. *Journal of Autism and Developmental Disorders, 29*, 439–484.

Fischer, K.W. & Rose, S.P. (1994). Dynamic development of coordination of components in brain and behavior: A framework for theory and research. In G. Dawson & K.W. Fischer (Eds.) *Human behavior and the developing brain.* (pp. 3–66) New York: Guilford Press.

Fombonne, E. (2003). Epidemiological surveys of autism and other pervasive developmental disorders: An update. *Journal of Autism and Developmental Disorders, 33, 365–382.*

Gresham, F.M. & MacMillan, D.L. (1997a). Autistic Recovery? An analysis and critique of the empirical evidence on the Early Intervention Project. *Behavioral Disorders, 22*, 185–201.

Gresham, F.M. & MacMillan, D.L. (1997b). Denial and defensiveness in the place of fact and reason: Rejoinder to Smith and Lovaas. *Behavioral Disorders, 22*, 219–230.

Guralnick, M.J. (1998). Effectiveness of early intervention for vulnerable children: A developmental perspective. *American Journal on Mental Retardation, 102*, 319–345.

Harris, S.L., & Handleman, J.S. (Eds.). (2001). *Preschool education programs for children with autism* (2ⁿᵈ ed.). Austin, TX: Pro-Ed.

Heflin, L.J. & Simpson, R.L. (1998). Interventions for children and youth with autism: Prudent choices in a world of exaggerated claims and empty promises. Part 1: Intervention and treatment option review. *Focus on Autism and Other Developmental Disabilities, 13*, 194–211.

Hurth, J., Shaw, E., Izeman, S.G., Whaley, K., & Rogers, S.J. (1999). Areas of agreement about effective practices among programs serving young children with autism spectrum disorders. *Infants and Young Children, 12*, 17–26.

Hwang, B., & Hughes, C. (2000). The effects of social interaction training on early social communicative skills of children with autism. *Journal of Autism and Developmental Disorders, 30*, 331-343.

Jordan, R., Jones, G., & Murray, D. (1998). Educational interventions for children with autism: A literature review of recent and current research (Report No. 77). London: Department for Education and Employment (Available from DfEE at http://www.dfes.gov.uk).

Kaiser, A.P. & Gray, D.B. (Eds.). (1993). *Enhancing children's communication: Research foundations for intervention.* Baltimore: Paul H. Brookes.

Lord, C. & Risi, S. (2000). Diagnosis of autism spectrum disorders in young children. In A.M. Wetherby and B.M. Prizant (Eds.), *Autism spectrum disorders: A transactional developmental perspective* (pp. 11–30). Baltimore: Paul Brookes.

Lovaas, O.I. (2002). *Teaching individuals with developmental delays: Basic intervention techniques.* Austin TX: Pro-Ed.

Maestro, S., Muratori, F., Cavallaro, M.C., Pei, F., Stern, D., Golse, B. et al. (2002). Attentional skills during the first 6 months of age in autism spectrum disorder. *Journal of the American Academy of Child & Adolescent Psychiatry, 41*, 1239–1245.

McConnell, S.R. (2002). Interventions to facilitate social interaction for young children with autism: Review of available research and recommendations for educational intervention and future research. *Journal of Autism and Developmental Disorders, 32*, 351–372.

Mundy, P. & Crowson, M. (1997). Joint attention and early social communication: Implications for research on intervention with autism. *Journal of Autism and Developmental Disorders, 27*, 653–676.

National Research Council. (2001). *Educating children with autism.* Committee on Educational Interventions with Children with Autism. Division of Behavioral and Social Sciences and Education. Washington, DC; National Academy Press.

Osterling, J.A., Dawson, G., & Munson, J.A. (2002). Early recognition of 1-year-old infants with autism spectrum disorder versus mental retardation. *Development and Psychopathology, 14*, 239–251.

Ramey, C.T. & Ramey, S.L. (1998). Early intervention and early experience. *American Psychologist, 53*, 109–120.

Rogers, S.J. (1998). Neuropsychology of autism in young children and its implications for early intervention. *Mental Retardation and Developmental Disabilities Research Reviews, 4*, 104–112.

Rogers, S.J. (2001). Diagnosis of autism before the age of 3. *International Review of Research in Developmental Disabilities, 23*, 1–31.

Rosenblatt, J., Bloom, P., & Koegel, R.L. (1995). Overselective responding: Description, implications, and intervention. In R.L. Koegel & L.K. Koegel (Eds.). *Teaching children with autism: Strategies for initiating positive interactions and improving learning opportunities.* (pp. 33–42). Baltimore: Paul H. Brookes.

Schopler, E., Reichler, R.J., Bashford, A., Lansing, M.D., & Marcus, L. M. (1990). *Psychoeducational Profile-Revised (PEP-R)*. Austin, TX: Pro-Ed.

Shea, V. (in press). A perspective on the research literature related to early intensive behavioral intervention (Lovaas) for young children with autism. *Autism*.

Smith, T. & Antolovich, M. (2000). Parental perceptions of supplemental interventions received by young children with autism in intensive behavior analytic treatment. *Behavioral Interventions, 15*, 83–97.

Smith, T. & Lovaas, O.I. (1997). The UCLA Young Autism Project: A reply to Gresham and MacMillan. *Behavioral Disorders, 22*, 202–218.

Strain, P.S. & Hoyson, M. (2000). The need for longitudinal, intensive social skill intervention: LEAP follow-up outcomes for children with autism. *Topics in Early Childhood Special Education, 20*, 116–122.

Trohanis, P. (2002). *Progress in providing services to young children with special needs and their families*. (NECTAS Notes No. 12). Chapel Hill: The University of North Carolina, FPG Child Development Institute, National Early Childhood Technical Assistance Center.

Wahlberg, T. (2001). The control theory of autism. In T. Wahlberg, F. Obiakor, S. Burkhardt, & A.F. Rotatori (Eds.), *Autism spectrum disorders: Educational and clinical intervention. Advances in special education*, Vol. 14 (pp. 19–35). Oxford: Elsevier Science Ltd.

Werner, E., Dawson, G., Osterling, J., & Dinno, N. (2000). Brief report: Recognition of autism spectrum disorder before one year of age: A retrospective study based on home videotapes. *Journal of Autism and Developmental Disorders, 30*, 157–162.

CHAPTER 11

Adult Services

INTRODUCTION

TEACCH's services for adults with autism spectrum disorders (ASD) are a natural extension of both the philosophy and methods that were originally developed for young children and their families (See Chapter 1, The Origins and History of the TEACCH Program). Starting in the late 1970's, TEACCH Centers began systematically expanding services for adolescents and adults with ASD. In recognition the life long impact of ASD, in 1979 the North Carolina legislature expanded the funding of TEACCH to include services to these older individuals and their families.

This chapter will review the history and literature on adult services for individuals with ASD, and then describe how TEACCH Centers have extended their traditional activities of diagnosis, treatment, and consultation to address the unique needs of adolescents and adults with ASD. The major focus of this chapter will be a description of two demonstration programs that serve as models for the successful application of TEACCH methods to both the residential and vocational services for adults—the Carolina Living and Learning Center (CLLC) and the TEACCH Supported Employment Program.

BACKGROUND LITERATURE

An appreciation in the literature for the life-long issues faced by individuals with ASD is relatively new. Schopler and Mesibov (1983) edited one of the first books to address the issues faced by adolescents and adults with ASD. Since then, there have been other excellent books by adults with ASD (e.g., Grandin, 1995; Williams, 1992), parents of adults with ASD (e.g., Parks, 2001), and professionals (e.g., Howlin, 1997) that chronicle the issues faced by adults with ASD.

Outcome studies, including Kanner's earliest work (Kanner & Eisenberg, 1956), Rutter's more systematic follow-up studies in the late 1960's (Lockyer &

Rutter, 1969, 1970, Rutter & Lockyer, 1967; Rutter, Greenfield, & Lockyer; 1967), Lotter's studies (Lotter, 1974a, 1974b) and that of Howlin, Goode, Hutton and Rutter (2004) have found variable outcomes for adults. Traditionally-cited best predictors of adult outcome have been early language and IQ scores (Howlin, 1997), although this finding is not universally accepted (Howlin et al., 2004). Further, most of these outcome studies pre-date the development of autism-specific services.

Because of limited recognition in the past of the lifelong implications of ASD, residential and vocational services for adults with ASD have been similarly limited. One factor that contributed to the lack of services for adults with ASD was that most residential and vocational training programs had been designed to serve individuals with mental retardation without ASD. As a result, these programs typically did not accept residents with ASD, or accepted them but had difficulty maintaining them in a program not specifically designed for their needs (Van Bourgondien & Reichle, 1997). Compared to individuals with developmental disabilities without ASD, adults with ASD were reported to have more difficulties with anxiety and agitation, ritualistic behaviors and the drive for sameness, social isolation, inappropriate social behaviors, self-stimulation, and atypical tempo that resulted in their moving at a slower pace than those around them (Everard, 1976; Kanner, Rodrigues & Ashenden, 1972, Mesibov, & Shea, 1980; Van Bourgondien, Mesibov & Castelloe, 1989). Several studies have found that individuals with ASD generally had behavior difficulties that required more time, effort, and different treatment approaches than approaches used with individuals with mental retardation alone (Mesibov & Shea, 1980; Van Bourgondien, Mesibov, & Castelloe, 1989; Van Bourgondien & Reichle, 1997).

Based on recognition of the different needs of individuals with ASD, residential programs specifically designed for individuals with ASD have been developed throughout the world (Giddan & Giddan, 1993; Van Bourgondien & Reichle, 1997). The impetus for most of these programs came from parents and teachers who were concerned about their children and students as they prepared to leave school.

Residential Programs

In 1990 when TEACCH's Carolina Living and Learning Center opened in North Carolina, there were only a few residential programs around the country specifically designed for individuals with ASD, such as Benhaven in Connecticut (Lettick, 1983; Simonson, Simonson, & Volkmar, 1990), the Jay Nolan Center in California (LaVigna, 1983), the Eden Family of Programs in New Jersey (Holmes, 1990; Holmes, 1997), and Community Services for Autistic Adults and Children in Maryland (CSAAC, 1995; Juhrs, 1988). There were also a small number of private, non-profit group homes specifically designed for individuals with ASD in North Carolina (Wall, 1990).

Vocational Programs

Vocational programming specifically designed for individuals with ASD has also been a relatively new area of services. Two approaches to providing appropriate day services are farming and employment in typical jobs in the community through supported employment programs.

Farming

Farming as a vocational activity for individuals with developmental disabilities is not a new concept. In the early 1900's, institutions in the United States frequently had a farming or gardening component. Although anecdotal evidence suggested that this physical activity was beneficial to the residents' health and general sense of well-being, the practice in the United States was discontinued because of human rights concerns and because of the economic impact, secondary to labor laws, of paying the residents for these activities.

However, in the past 30 years farming programs have become a relatively common phenomenon in European countries such as England, France, and Denmark (Giddan & Giddan, 1993). In 1974, Somerset Court was started as the first community for adults with ASD in England (Giddan & Giddan, 1993; Van Bourgondien & Elgar, 1990). Ny Allergard in Denmark was founded in 1983 by a group of parents and professionals (Giddan & Giddan, 1993). These programs, which emphasize farming and landscaping as vocational activities, are located in communities where these are also the common occupations of the neurotypical population. Another program, Bittersweet Farms outside Toledo, Ohio was started in 1982 based on the model of Somerset Court and on the classroom experience of the founder, Bettye Ruth Kay (Kay, 1990).

Proponents of these farming communities indicate that the benefits include increased motivation and satisfaction as the workers engage in meaningful activities, reduced behavior problems as a result of the emphasis on physical activity, and greater consistency in teaching appropriate social and communication skills in settings that have integrated living and work environments (Giddan & Giddan, 1993; Kay, 1990; Van Bourgondien & Reichle, 2001). Another advantage of agriculture and landscaping programs is that they include a wide variety of functional and meaningful outdoor tasks at different developmental levels. Individuals with ASD with very basic skills as well as more able individuals can all participate in meaningful ways, from clearing the land and providing mulch, to planting and harvesting, to involvement in related community integration projects such as small businesses (e.g., greenhouse, engine repair shop), mobile landscaping crews, or farmers' markets. These rural programs emphasize the same goals as vocational programs located in more urban settings—maximizing the quality of life and increasing skills and independence at home and in the larger community (Van Bourgondien & Reichle, 1997).

Supported Employment

The Developmental Disabilities Act of 1984 (PL 98-527) defined Supported Employment as employment that (a) is for people with developmental disabilities for whom competitive employment at or above the minimum wage is unlikely and who, because of their disabilities, need intensive on-going support to perform in a work setting; (b) is conducted in a variety of settings, particularly worksites in which people without disabilities are employed; and (c) is supported by any activity needed to sustain paid work by persons with disabilities, including supervision, training, and transportation (Federal Register, 1984; Keel, Mesibov, & Woods, 1997). The Rehabilitation Act Amendments of 1986 (PL 99-506) and 1992 (PL 102-569) contained similar language, and contributed to the establishment of funding streams for various supported employment services.

Earlier efforts in supported employment had demonstrated that individuals with mental retardation could earn wages in a competitive work force (Rusch & Mithaug, 1980; Sowers, Thompson, and Connis, 1979; Wehman, 1981). Successful supported employment efforts for the general population of individuals with development disabilities were documented by Wehman and colleagues (Wehman et al., 1985), who introduced procedures for providing training and support for individuals with disabilities *at the job site.* Another important aspect of their work was the assessment and matching of the individual to the worksite. Providing training and assistance with activities around work such as transportation and interviewing for the job were other essential elements of their approach.

During the 1980's, in part because of governmental support, the number of programs and services developed to integrate individuals with disabilities into community settings increased dramatically (Goldberg, McLean, LaVigna, Fratolillo, & Sullivan, 1990). Between 1986 and 1989, 1400 programs were authorized by state agencies to provide supported employment (Schafer, Wehman, Kregel & West, 1990).

Research in the late 1980's indicated that the majority of individuals being served in integrated supported employment settings were people with mental retardation with mild to moderate disabilities. People with ASD have typically had more limited options for integrated employment (Keel, Mesibov, & Woods, 1997). For example, Ballaban-Gil, Rapin, Tuchman, & Shinnar (1996) found only 11% of a broad sample of adults with ASD employed in typical community jobs. In other studies, even among the most able individuals with ASD, fewer than one quarter were employed (Howlin, 1997; Howlin et al., 2004).

TEACCH began its formal Supported Employment program in 1989 as a collaborative effort with the Autism Society of North Carolina and the North Carolina Vocational Rehabilitation Services. Another program, Community Services for Autistic Adults and Children in Rockville, Maryland (CSAAC, 1995; Smith, Belcher, & Juhrs, 1995) has also specialized in employment services for people with ASD with severe disabilities. Utilizing behavioral techniques, that program has demonstrated how to decrease behavior problems and increase production rates in individuals they served (Smith & Coleman, 1986). The use of supported employment techniques with people with ASD in Great Britain has been described by Howlin (1997). In a 1999 study, Mawhood and Howlin compared the outcome for participants with ASD in a supported employment program specifically designed for people with ASD with the outcome for similar adults who did not have specialized supported employment services. Results demonstrated that the employment rate and job levels of program participants were higher than those of controls, as were number of hours worked and wages. Although the costs of this program were high, they significantly reduced over the two years of the study.

EFFECTIVENESS OF
TREATMENT PROGRAMS

The effectiveness of both residential and vocational programs for adults with ASD is based on careful assessments that include information about the individual's strengths and interests, as well as the use of adaptive techniques that increase the individual's understanding of the world, independence, and social skills.

Residential and vocational programs that have been specifically designed for individuals with ASD (Holmes, 1990; LaVigna, 1983; Lettick, 1983; Meyer, 2001; Smith, Belcher, & Juhrs, 1995; Wall, 1990) have emphasized the importance of understanding the unique learning style of each individual with ASD. Individualized supports should be based on a detailed assessment of the adult's interests, skills, and needs (Mesibov, Troxler, & Boswell, 1988). Adults with ASD, like children with ASD, generally do not function well without individualized support services that recognize their idiosyncratic style of understanding their environments, learning, and behaving (see Chapter 3, The Culture of Autism).

For assessment results to be helpful, it is important to identify more than just the individual's deficits (Van Bourgondien & Schopler, 1996). Recognizing the person's strengths, interests, emerging skills, and work habits will have a greater impact on the development of treatment objectives and teaching strategies than merely knowing what the person cannot do. Utilizing the interests and preferences of individuals with ASD has been shown to increase their morale in leisure activities (Favell & Cannon, 1976), spontaneous verbal requests (Dyer, 1989) and motivation in work situations (Van Bourgondien & Woods, 1992). LeBlanc, Schroeder, and Mayo (1997) have suggested that focusing on strengths and interests can also provide direction for securing jobs for individuals with ASD.

The CLLC and Supported Employment Program utilize the Structured Teaching techniques that were originally developed by TEACCH for children at school and at home (Schopler, Mesibov, & Hearsey, 1995; see also Chapter 4,

Structured Teaching). Utilizing the visual strengths of individuals with ASD involves physical organization, schedules, work/activity system, and a variety of visual and organizational strategies for clarifying task requirements. As reviewed by Mesibov, Browder and Kirkland (2002), previous research has shown the effectiveness of using schedules to ease transitions (Dooley, Wilczenski, & Torem, 2001; Flannery & Horner, 1994), to increase independence in task performance (Anderson, Sherman, Sheldon, & McAdam, 1997; Krantz, MacDuff, & McClannahan, 1993; Pierce & Schriebman, 1994), to follow a preset work or school routine (Browder & Minarovic, 2000; Clarke, Dunlap, & Vaughn, 1999; Hall, McClannahan, & Krantz, 1995), and to increase the initiation, length, and generalization of leisure activities (Bambara & Ager, 1992; MacDuff, Krantz, & McClannahan, 1993). In addition, the use of visual strategies provides predictability, thus reducing confusion and behavior problems (Clarke et al., 1999; Dooley et al., 2001; Flannery & Horner, 1994, Krantz et al., 1993). The effectiveness of the use of schedules has been demonstrated in classrooms, group homes, family homes, work settings, and in the community (Mesibov et al., 2002).

TEACCH CENTERS—SERVICES FOR
ADULTS WITH ASD

The extension of services to adolescent and adults was a natural evolution of the TEACCH's work with children. Research demonstrated that the Childhood Autism Rating Scale (CARS; Schopler, Reichler, Devellis, & Daly, 1980; Schopler, Reichler, & Renner, 1988) was also a reliable and valid diagnostic instrument for adolescents and adults, although the cut-off for autism was found to be 2.2 points lower (Mesibov, Schopler, Schaffer, & Michal, 1984; Schopler & Mesibov, 1983). To assist with the transition from schools to vocational settings, the Adolescent and Adult Psychoeducational Profile (AAPEP) was developed (Mesibov, Schopler, Schaffer, & Landrus, 1989). A criterion-referenced measurement tool, the AAPEP assesses functioning in six areas—independence, communication, leisure, social, vocational skills, and vocational behaviors. Through direct observation as well as interviews with school/work personnel and caregivers, the AAPEP has been demonstrated to be an effective tool for generating treatment objectives. In recognition of the increasing diversity in both the population of individuals with ASD as well as the expanding vocational options, a revised version of the AAPEP (to be called the TEACCH Transition Assessment Profile [TTAP]) is in the process of development.

Parent training sessions are also offered to parents of adolescents and adults (see Chapter 8, Parents). Consultation to other agencies, a traditional TEACCH function, has been expanded to include work with staff members from vocational and day programs for adults with ASD, as well as a variety of residential support programs.

Follow-up studies of adults with ASD have indicated an increase in social interest and awareness with age (Rutter, 1970; Mesibov, 1983). Therefore, an increased emphasis on teaching social skills is appropriate for the older age groups. The TEACCH Centers provide consultation to high school special education classrooms that include social development as part of the curriculum. For adolescents who are in integrated classroom settings, the centers either provide social skill groups or work with other professionals in their geographic area to develop groups (see Chapter 7, Social Skills).

For adolescents and adults who are more verbal, individual counseling sessions are offered. These sessions frequently focus on helping clients understand ASD and how it affects their learning style and behavior. Sessions are individualized to help the person address issues such as age-appropriate self-care skills (e.g., money management) and developing coping skills, problem-solving skills, or social skills. Developing social cognition (that is, understanding what others are thinking and expecting in social situations) is one aspect of developing social skills.

Overall, Structured Teaching (see Chapter 4, Structured Teaching) is applicable to all adult services, although assessment and treatment strategies can take a different form when integrated into adult residential and vocational settings. To illustrate the use of TEACCH concepts with adults, the rest of this chapter will focus on TEACCH's model residential and vocational programs.

THE CAROLINA LIVING AND
LEARNING CENTER

The Carolina Living and Learning Center (CLLC) is located on a 79-acre farm, where staff members and clients work collaboratively to perform the various functions of the home and the farm. The mission of the CLLC is to maximize the quality of life of the adults with ASD who live and work there and to help them engage in productive, meaningful activities in both the residential and vocational settings. As a treatment setting, the CLLC was designed to provide residential and vocational training to adults with ASD in a manner that best suits the interests, strengths, and abilities of each individual. Its goal is to teach the residents and day students new skills in all areas of development that they can use as independently as possible. As a component of the University of North Carolina—Chapel Hill, the CLLC has as a secondary objective investigating and demonstrating the effectiveness of the TEACCH treatment model.

Background and Rationale

In the early 1980's, the North Carolina Mental Health Study Commission conducted a survey to assess the service needs of the adults with ASD in the state. Of the 393 people located, most were at home with their families, 10% were in institutions, and fewer than 15% were in group homes. No more than 50% were in day programs (or still in school if they were between 18 and 21 years). Based on the lack of appropriate community-based programs identified in this survey, the Mental Health Study Commission recommended to the North Carolina Legislature that funding be provided to expand the services for adults with ASD in North Carolina. As a result of that recommendation and with ongoing collaboration with Autism Society of North Carolina, the development of the CLLC was initiated in 1983.

When the CLLC opened in 1990, there were three major objectives for this demonstration program (Van Bourgondien & Reichle, 1996). The first objective was to develop another option on the continuum of services for individuals with ASD. Unlike the few existing group homes for adults with ASD, this model integrated residential and vocational programming within the same site and administrative structure. This combination of residential and vocational training was designed to provide greater consistency in teaching new skills and in preventing and managing behavior problems throughout the entire day. The second objective was to extend the model of collaboration, previously developed with professionals and parents (Schopler, Mesibov, Shigley, & Bashford, 1984), to include direct collaboration between residents with ASD and staff members in maintaining a farm. Finally, because the CLLC is part of the University of North Carolina - Chapel Hill, the third objective was to develop a demonstration site where Structured Teaching strategies originally developed for children could be adapted and evaluated in a residential setting for adults. The results of this research could then be incorporated into training programs for professionals working in a variety of residential and vocational settings.

Program Description

Participants

The CLLC serves 15 adults with ASD who live in two neighboring homes (five adults in one home and ten in the other home). There are also up to 5 day students who participate to varying degrees in the day program. Some of these day students work as much as 40 hours a week on the farm while others are high school students who come one day a week as a job sampling experience.

Residents come from across the state of North Carolina and must be at least 18 years of age at admission. The current residents range in age from 28 to 46 years old. There are 13 men and 2 women, with a range of verbal abilities from non-verbal to varying degrees of functional speech. All the residents have moderate to severe ASD and have significant behavioral and/or adaptive challenges that require twenty-four hour per day supervision. Their intellectual difficulties range from significant learning difficulties to severe mental retardation. A number of the residents have additional medical or psychiatric diagnoses including hearing loss, seizures, or psychiatric difficulties such as affective disorder, obsessive-compulsive disorder, bi-polar disorder, and atypical psychosis.

Selecting clients for community-based treatment homes like the CLLC is a challenge (Van Bourgondien & Reichle, 1997). One the one hand, there is a very large population of applicants with severe disabilities and intense behavioral problems and supervision needs, with understandably desperate families. On the other hand, the literature suggests that the best way to optimize the learning and living experience for the individuals with ASD is to have a balance of skill levels, behavioral problems, and supervision needs among the residents (LaVigna, 1983, Wall, 1990). Selecting a group of residents with a variety of skills and behaviors not only helps ensure an individualized educational experience for each resident, but it also contributes to the prevention of burnout in staff members who work for long periods of time without breaks (Van Bourgondien & Schopler, 1990; Wall, 1990). The CLLC residents were chosen from applicants who were in the greatest need of appropriate residential and vocational services, with the potential residents' self-care and independence skills and their level of behavioral difficulties also taken into account. The extent to which potential residents were interested in and capable of participation in a vocational program that involved farming and landscaping was also an important consideration.

Curriculum

The emphasis of both the work and living programs is to teach the worker/resident new skills that he or she can use as independently as possible on the farm, at home, and in the community. During the course of the day, an individual resident experiences a balance of activities that include (a) formalized teaching activities; (b) independent tasks; and (c) apprentice activities performed in partnership with staff members.

Individualized treatment goals are the backbone of the program. The formal treatment programs are designed to teach functional and meaningful activities that can be integrated into the person's day-to-day life. Systematic teaching strategies and data collection procedures provide consistency and the means of evaluating the effectiveness of the behavioral and skill training programs. Both incidental teaching (McGee, Almeida, Sulzer-Azaroff & Feldman, 1992) and Structured Teaching strategies (see Chapter 4, Structured Teaching) are important aspects of the program. Clients are actively involved in all activities and encouraged to do things for themselves including personal hygiene/dressing, household chores, meal preparation, laundry, vocational activities, exercise, recreation/leisure activities, and community involvement.

The residential and vocational direct care staff members play a variety of roles. The staff member sets up the visual structures—the schedule, work/activity systems, and visual instructions that enable the person with ASD to function as independently as possible. The staff member is a teacher of new skills utilizing the formal teaching program strategies. The staff member also works performing the tasks the client may not be able to do yet, or serving as a model for how to do a given task. Just as collaboration between parents and professionals is an important ingredient in work with children with ASD (Schopler, et al., 1984), this direct collaboration between clients and staff members is an important aspect of the program. Utilizing an apprenticeship model, staff members work along side the workers with ASD in all aspects of farming and landscaping.

Assessment

At the CLLC, ongoing assessment of the skills, interests, behaviors, and needs of the adults with ASD is an integral part of both the vocational and residential programs. In addition, as part of the annual review, each individual's cognitive, communication, social, and adaptive skills (self-care, domestic and community) are re-assessed to determine their progress and to establish treatment goals for the upcoming year. Vocational skills are also assessed; the assessment includes workers' knowledge of the tools and equipment utilized in farming, landscaping and baking as well as the specific skills involved in each area.

Vocational Curriculum Areas

Gardening

There are numerous flower, herb, and vegetable gardens throughout the property, so gardening and landscaping operations provide a variety of work opportunities. All tasks are taught and carried out using Structured Teaching methods (see Chapter 4, Structured Teaching) including the use of an individualized schedule and work/activity system that show the worker where to go, what work to do, how much work to do, how to see progress and 'finished' and what to do next.

The simplest tasks include work filling seed cells and trays with soil mix, and packaging 1 to 3 seeds into film canisters using a visual jig or diagram. (Prepackaging the seeds helps to assure evenly distributed planting of seeds at a later step in the process.) Slightly more difficult tasks include planting seeds in flats (use of a jig and a funnel helps to assure proper seed depth in soil), fertilizing, and watering flats.

Planting strategies for the greenhouse can be generalized to planting in the garden. The individual may use a jig, picture, or written system to obtain the tools necessary to plant, then use a "destination card" to locate the correct garden in which to plant, and then find a series of rings in the garden marking where to plant the previously packaged seeds. Tape may be placed by a supervisor on a seed planting tool to indicate the appropriate depth for particular seeds, to prevent errors of planting too shallow or too deep. The individual knows exactly how much work is to occur before a break because he or she can see the number of seed canisters and can watch their number dwindle as the empty canisters go into a "finished" bucket.

Watering tasks are set up so that over- and under-watering are less likely to occur. Flags, markers, or hoops may be placed beside or around the plants to be watered. The individual may transport 5- or 10-gallon buckets to the garden and use a specific number of scoops of water on each plant before removing the flag or marker. The individual can recognize that the job is finished when all the flags have been removed.

The seemingly endless chore of weeding may be clarified by the use of hoops to designate specific areas to be weeded. Plants to be saved within the hoop can be covered by soda or milk bottles so that the individual can succeed in weeding without error. The use of a chip system to help the client water or weed a specific number of hoops before a break is also helpful.

Elements of several of the systems already mentioned can also be used in the mulching, compost layering, fertilizing, and chipping of organic matter for the gardens or landscaping. Each of these tasks involves providing workers with the visual structure they need to gather their own tools, go to the proper garden, obtain the organic material, place it in the desired location, and know when they have completed the activity.

Landscaping

A primary goal of the landscaping program is the upkeep and management of the CLLC grounds so that the environment is attractive and pleasant for clients, staff members, and visitors. The activities of the landscaping crew involve mowing, raking, weeding, planting flowers or trees, pruning, edging, and fertilizing lawns and shrubs. Visual structure is utilized to help the landscaper with ASD know how and where to perform a particular activity (cones for mowing or raking, hoops for weeding, etc.).

Another goal is for the clients to generalize landscaping skills learned at the farm to other settings in the community, including customers' home yards and a local camp. In addition to the previously mentioned landscaping jobs, the landscaping activities performed in community settings include applying mulch/compost, removing unwanted branches or brush, creating walking paths, and sweeping walks, patios, and driveways.

Baking/Food Preparation

The baking curriculum has many of the same benefits as the farming program. The task of making food is meaningful to the residents, and the process can be broken down into very concrete tasks at a variety of skill levels. The primary baking activities involve baking bread and rolls for consumption in the home. Visual systems are used to help identify ingredients and utensils as well as the steps in the baking process.

Benefits of the Vocational Program for Clients

Most CLLC clients could not be maintained in previous day placements because of their behaviors, so all of the clients have experienced an increase in participation in meaningful day activities since coming to the CLLC. Clients who work in the farm and landscaping programs are paid for their work based on their productivity and rate of completion compared to a typical person completing the same task. For the majority of clients, income from wages has increased relative to what they earned before coming to the CLLC. Monthly income varies greatly across residents because of variability in their skills and performance; in addition, residents' earnings can vary from month to month because of the seasonal nature of certain tasks (e.g., mowing) and because of fluctuations in behavior and subsequent productivity.

Residential Program

The CLLC is both the residents' home and a treatment center designed to utilize individuals' strengths and interests in order to address their needs. The curriculum in the residential program (evening and weekends) emphasizes maximizing the involvement of residents in taking care of their own personal and household needs, developing and maintaining leisure, recreational, and social skills based on their interests, and generalizing a variety of skills to community settings. Daily domestic activities range from the personal hygiene, dressing, and laundry activities to chores related to preparing meals and cleaning/maintaining bedrooms and shared living areas.

After work each day, the residents are likely to engage in one of three activities, typically meal preparation, community outings, or exercise. Residents from each home take turns being responsible for the preparation of all meals. The goals are for the men and women to participate in all aspects of meal preparation and for them to learn to do as much of the preparation as independently as possible. For aspects of meal preparation that a resident is not yet ready to learn, he or she is involved as an apprentice/helper.

Residents not involved in meal preparation on a given afternoon may be involved in doing errands in the community, e.g., grocery shopping, banking, post office, therapy appointments, haircuts, shopping for clothes or personal needs. Alternatively, the residents may participate in an exercise activity either on the farm or in the community.

After dinner, residents are engaged in typical clean-up chores and personal hygiene activities. In addition, special evening times are set aside to work on communication skills, developing leisure interests, and social skills.

Developing Independence through Visual Structure

Schedules

Each resident has an individualized daily schedule that helps him or her understand the sequence of the day and where he/she will go next. The schedules involve the use of written words, pictures, photos or objects; the decision about the level of abstraction to use is based not on an individual's highest skill level when calm, organized, and focused, but on the person's level of conceptual understanding and literacy on his or her worst days. The rationale for this is that many individuals with ASD demonstrate great variability in their processing skills, and we want to be sure that they can understand their schedules and anticipate what will be happening especially on the days where their skills may be diminished.

Most residents' schedules are located in the hallway of their homes and in their primary work setting (barn, potting shed, or greenhouse). Several residents have portable schedules that they carry with them throughout the day. A few residents are still learning to understand the concepts involved in schedules, and are on object transition systems where the staff members present the object signifying the next activity directly to the residents. (See Chapter 6, Communication, for more information).

Work/Activity Systems

All program participants have individualized work/activity systems or "to do lists" that help them understand (1) what activity to do; (2) how much to do; (3) how to know they are making progress and when they are finished; (4) what is going to happen next. All residents have work/activity systems conveniently located in the kitchen, bathroom, exercise room, and bedrooms as well as the barn, potting shed, or other locations where they engage in structured activities. These systems are used for helping the residents independently complete hygiene tasks, domestic chores, leisure activities, and work tasks. The staff member sets up the work/activity system at the beginning of each activity. The work/activity systems may consist of written lists of activities, word cards, picture cards, number or color cards, or left to right basket systems, depending on the level of conceptual understanding of each individual.

Visual Instructions

Within each of the various domestic, leisure, and work activities, residents often need additional information or instructions for how to complete the activity independently. Written lists, picture/word, or picture lists can help some clients know how to clean their room, make a meal, play a game, plant a bulb, etc. For other residents, organizing materials with the use of containers, labeling materials with picture or color cues, or using outline jigs can increase their understanding of what needs to be done with a given task.

Expressive Communication

Anecdotal reports by parents of adults with ASD (Howlin, 1997; Van Bourgondien & Schopler, 1996) suggest that as individuals with ASD leave school and enter adult day programs, many have difficulty generalizing previously learned expressive communication skills to new settings that do not put as much emphasis on teaching expressive skills. One advantage of the twenty-four hour a day nature of the CLLC is that communication programs designed to increase the initiation and use of expressive communication systems are consistently used throughout the day. Utilizing TEACCH communication principles (See Chapter 6, Communication), each client is assessed to determine what mode of expressive communication is most meaningful—objects, gestures, pictures, written words, sign language, or verbalizations.

Elliot, Hall and Soper's (1991) research on teaching language to adults with ASD and mental retardation found that even in a test situation biased toward analog teaching (that is, discrete trials in a controlled setting), natural language teaching is a very effective way of facilitating the generalization and retention of new language skills. Consistent with this finding, the CLLC looks for natural opportunities throughout the day to teach and practice expressive communication skills.

At the most basic level, residents are taught to request what they want to eat or what leisure activity they would like to do. Once individuals have become familiar with the options and have been taught how to make a choice, choice boards for snacks, free time, and community activities are utilized. (The visual cues to assist with requesting are portable to enable generalization to community settings.) More advanced communication skills being taught include learning to ask for help and learning to ask to leave a difficult situation instead of having a behavioral outburst. Even for verbal individuals, some type of visual reminder of things to say (such as a picture or a written reminder to get the attention of the other person before making a request) helps them to utilize expressive language more consistently.

The teaching strategies utilized in this area of the curriculum are also consistent with Quill's work (1998) and the Picture Exchange Communication System (Bondy & Frost, 1994) approach to teaching expressive communication skills to individuals with ASD.

Leisure and Social Skill Training

Leisure skills are important for several reasons. First, problems with staying appropriately engaged during free time distinguish adults with ASD from adults with other developmental disabilities in residential settings (Van Bourgondien et al., 1989), whereas leisure skills enable people with ASD to entertain themselves safely and appropriately. Second, shared leisure interests are the basis for social relationships even among neurotypical people, and can be for people with ASD also.

The CLLC provides opportunities for the residents to acquire new leisure skills using the schedules, work systems, and visual instructions that have been demonstrated to increase variety of leisure activities and self initiation (Bambara & Ager, 1992) and to increase response chains and the generalization of these skills (MacDuff et al., 1993). In addition to individualized teaching programs designed to increase these skills, the entire CLLC program has at least one evening a week specifically devoted to teaching new leisure skills. In order to increase the motivation to engage in these activities (Favell & Cannon, 1976), activities are adapted to include the special interests of the residents (e.g., Newscaster lotto, Exit sign puzzles).

The development of social skills at the CLLC is a continuous and integrated goal of the program. At the most basic level, the development of social skills is

naturally integrated into both residential and vocational activities by simultaneously involving more than one client in the same activity in the same location.
Residents vary in the level of social interaction that is most appropriate. For
some, an appropriate goal is just learning to share space and be in proximity to
another person (sit at the same table, or work in the same garden). Others may
be ready for some simple sharing or turn-taking. Before combining residents for
an activity, each individual is individually taught how to do the activity, such
as raking leaves or playing bingo. Then when residents do the activity together,
the only new element being taught is how to do the task with another person
present.

The residents participate in a number of formal "social club" activities
designed to increase their social skills around recreational and leisure activities.
Weekly social clubs meetings, when residents are divided into small groups
based on their skills and interests, are held at the CLLC one night a week. While
the activities vary from week to week and from group to group, a common goal
of all groups is to teach the residents to initiate a trade or swap with another
person, because the inability to initiate an exchange with another person is a
deficit that was seen in all residents with ASD regardless of their other abilities.
Making a purchase, communicating a shoe size to get bowling shoes, giving
someone a ticket to gain admission, and handing someone a library card to
get a book are basic community skills that all involve trading something to get
something. First teaching this initiation through role play and practice sessions
at home prepares both the residents and staff members for generalizing these
skills to the community.

A number of residents also participate in social groups in the community
where they can interact with peers with whom they don't live. Some of these
groups are designed for specific clientele—a friendship group for individuals
who have ASD and are deaf, a woman's group, a social skills group for individuals with high functioning ASD, a church group, etc.

As with all areas of curriculum, each resident has individually identified
social skill goals that may involve a variety of teaching strategies from role play,
picture/written prompts, social scripts, or social stories.

Behavior Management

The CLLC emphasizes a preventative approach to behavior problems. When
the reasons behind a behavior are understood, sources of stress that may be
contributing to the behavior can be decreased or eliminated, and strategies can
be utilized to teach the person what to do instead of the inappropriate behavior.

A major component of preventing behavior problems are the schedules,
work/activity systems, and visual instructions that help to reduce confusion
and make life more predictable for the individual with ASD. Researchers have
found that using schedules to make transitions (Dooley et al., 2001; Flannery &
Horner, 1994) and using picture activity lists to let the individual know what to
do (Clarke, Dunlap & Vaughn, 1999) have decreased behavior problems.

In addition, the use of augmentative communication systems reduces frustration and increases the individual's ability to make choices and indicate preferences. Providing individuals with severe handicaps the opportunity to choose from a variety of activities has been demonstrated to increase motivation and decrease behavior problems (Dyer, Dunlap, & Winterling, 1990; Favell & Cannon, 1976).

Exercise, both in the farming activities and in the recreational curriculum, also plays a role in decreasing stress and behavior difficulties. Kay (1990) anecdotally reports a similar finding at Bittersweet Farm. Controlled studies have also found aerobic exercise to have beneficial effects in reducing maladaptive behaviors and increasing on-task behaviors for individuals with ASD (Allison, Basele, & MacDonald, 1991; Elliot, Dobbin, Rose, & Soper, 1994; McGimsey & Favell, 1985; Rosenthal-Malek & Mitchell, 1997). At the CLLC, the daily work activities on the farm involve a great deal of physical activity as the workers move about the acres carrying equipment and gardening materials. In addition, recreational activities including opportunities for hiking, swimming, and riding bicycles are dispersed throughout the week and weekend.

Another stress reduction activity for some individuals at the CLLC is systematic relaxation (Cautela & Groden, 1978) which combines breathing, tensing and relaxing muscle, and some guided imagery.

More traditional behavior plans, such as behavioral contracts or reinforcement schedules using the interests of the person with ASD, may also be employed. These plans, involving 'first desired behavior, then high-interest activity' sequences, highlight and support the social rules or behavioral expectations.

About half of the residents at the CLLC take medication to address psychiatric symptoms or behaviors. In all cases, medication use is integrated with a behavior plan that emphasizes the reduction in problem behaviors through a preventative intervention approach. The behavioral progress of all residents is monitored through on-going data collection and charting.

Role of Families

Even though the residents are adults, their families continue to play a major role in their treatment planning and social lives. The specific roles family members play in the life of their adult son or daughter vary with the individual needs and preferences of the family. Some families maintain a very active role in decision-making about their adult child's treatment plan, much as they did when their child lived at home and attended school. These parents participate at least yearly in formal meetings about their son or daughter, and they also collaborate with the staff members more informally throughout the year. Other families have switched their focus to emphasizing their role as more of a social/recreational outlet for their son or daughter, taking them home on weekends or holidays. Staff members work with the families to help promote the level and type of involvement that seems to work best for the person with ASD and their family members.

Communication and collaboration between families and the staff members at the CLLC is promoted through regular phone calls and through contact books that accompany the client home on visits, as well as through formal written reports each year. Families have at least yearly opportunities to meet individually with the treatment team. In addition, there are quarterly family meetings where the CLLC families come together as a group with administrative staff members to review and discuss program-wide issues.

The type of direct communication between the adult with ASD and his or her family members depends to a great extent on the communication skills of the person with ASD. All residents participate in a weekly letter-writing activity where cards or letters are made to send home to family members. The involvement of the individual with ASD could be typing a message into a template on the computer, dictating a message for a staff member to write, copying a dot-to-dot message that was written by a helper, or selecting a picture of himself or herself engaged in an activity to send along with a note written by a staff member. Family members report that they enjoy reading these letters about the resident's weekly activities. Some residents also have regular phone contact with family members.

Program Evaluation

The effectiveness of the CLLC's treatment program was evaluated in a study (Van Bourgondien, Reichle, & Schopler, 2003) that compared the programming and progress of the first 6 residents at the CLLC with that of 26 other adults who lived in other settings (group homes = 10, institutions = 6, and family homes = 10). The participants were placed into the CLLC treatment condition by a 'systematic, fair assignment process' originally developed by Landesman (1987). Eligible applicants to the CLLC were matched into three groups based on cognitive abilities, communication skills, degree of ASD, overall level of behavioral difficulties, and need for supervision. Two participants from each group were admitted to the CLLC (N = 6) based on part-random, part-clinical assignment procedure. (Not only was this procedure helpful in making sure the treatment group was representative of the population from which it was sampled, but it also helped family members feel that this provided a fair selection process.)

The study compared the behaviors, skills, and treatment programming of the 32 participants 6 months prior to the opening of the CLLC, at admission, and at 6 months and 12 months after admission.

Results indicated that the participants who moved into the CLLC experienced a higher quality of treatment than the participants in the control settings. Compared to both their own baseline and to the control groups, the participants in the CLLC experienced a significant increase in the presence of structure and individualized programming in the areas of communication and social skill development, the use of visual systems to promote independence, the use of developmental planning, and the use of positive, preventative behavior management strategies. The CLLC was also rated by the researchers who visited the program as a more desirable place to live, and the CLLC families were significantly more satisfied than the control families. Based on exploratory analyses of all 32 participants, the use of the TEACCH Structured Teaching concepts over time was related to a decrease in behavior difficulties.

TEACCH SUPPORTED
EMPLOYMENT PROGRAM

The mission of the Supported Employment (SE) Program is to provide a stable and predictable work environment where the person with ASD can, as independently as possible, be a contributing member of the work force. The benefits of supported employment to the person with ASD range from the direct benefits of increased wages and engagement in meaningful and valued employment, to the more indirect benefits of integration in work settings with neurotypical employees. Employees with ASD increase their sense of self-worth, and at the same time increase public awareness of the skills and potential of people with ASD. The community also benefits from the decreased cost of governmental support to the competitively employed individual.

Background and Rationale

As mentioned previously, the TEACCH mandate was expanded in 1979 to include services to adolescents and adults with ASD and their families. In that same year, the first adult with ASD was placed in a part-time job at a University of North Carolina—Chapel Hill library with a job coach. This first placement and others that soon followed were precipitated in part by the difficulties these adults experienced in sheltered workshops that were designed for people with mental retardation without ASD. The physical settings of sheltered workshops, which included large numbers of people, open spaces, noise, and visual distractions, were sources of stress to many individuals with ASD. In contrast, community settings could be individualized based on the strengths, interests, sensory needs, and need for structure of the prospective employee.

The informal supported employment efforts of the TEACCH program in North Carolina in the early 1980's paralleled the nationwide moment to develop such services. TEACCH's formal Supported Employment program began in 1989 in collaboration with the Autism Society of North Carolina and the North Carolina Vocational Rehabilitation Services.

Program Description

Participants

Since the SE program was formally established in the 1989, more than 200 individuals with ASD have been placed in jobs in the community. Some of the individuals placed in jobs had been TEACCH clients for many years, while many others were specifically referred to the SE program by parents, sheltered workshops, North Carolina Vocational Rehabilitation Services, or other individuals and agencies. Currently the workers with ASD range in age from 18 to 56 years, and the majority (>85%) are men. In addition to the diagnosis of ASD, most individuals also have some intellectual difficulties; their intelligence scores range from profound mental retardation to significantly above average, with most clients in the mildly mentally retardation to low average range.

Acceptance in the SE program has been based on a variety of factors including the individual's skills and behaviors, and potential funding sources. SE staff members assess whether the individual might benefit from Supported Employment by meeting with the potential client, observing the individual in a workshop or classroom setting, reviewing previous evaluation reports, and meeting with families or residential program staff members.

Overview of Program

In an effort to provide the most appropriate and individualized program possible for each client, TEACCH utilizes four different models of Supported Employment—the One-to-One model, the Mobile Crew model, the Shared Support model, and the Independent model. These models differ only in the amount of support provided to the employee with ASD. Within each model of support, there is an emphasis on assessing in order to utilize the individual's strengths and interests, identifying appropriate jobs and settings, applying Structured Teaching techniques, collaborating with families/caregivers and employers, providing necessary long-term support services, and insuring an appropriate job match in which the employee, the employer, and family/caregiver are all satisfied.

Each of the models incorporates the use of 'job coaches' employed by TEACCH, who provide on-going support for a person or groups of people with ASD. Based on the results of careful assessment, job coaches help clients find jobs and then use the Structured Teaching principles to teach clients the necessary vocational skills, behaviors, and social skills for the employment setting. The job coach is also available to assist clients with completing tasks and to accommodate for fluctuating job performance, in order to insure the accuracy and quality of completed work. If clients become overwhelmed or frustrated, the job coach assists with stress reduction strategies, which help the client to remain calm and focused, and to attend better to job responsibilities. Job coaches also educate co-workers and supervisors about ASD, and act as liaisons between the individuals with ASD and their employers.

Models of Support

One-to-One Model

The One-to-One model of supported employment consists of one job coach and one person with ASD. A company in the community employs the individual with ASD, and the job coach is located on-site throughout the entire workday. Because of the availability of a job coach to provide individualized job training and support, employees can be maintained in a wide variety of jobs that maximize the individuals' strengths and interests.

The biggest difference between clients in this service model and the other models is the intense support these clients require. To meet this need, the job coach is present to adapt and modify structure as often as necessary for the individual to be successful. This may include setting up or changing schedules and visual cues in the work environment throughout the day. Also, people with ASD who work in this model tend to have poorer communication skills and coping strategies; therefore, the job coach spends time acting as a liaison between the person with ASD and the employer. This ensures that everyone clearly understands each other's expectations, opinions, and ideas.

Mobile Crew Model

For those individuals who require less intensive support than the One-to-One model, there is the Mobile Crew. The Mobile Crew Model of supported employment consists of one job coach and two to three clients with ASD. The types of services the Mobile Crew provides currently include home cleaning and landscaping. The job coach remains with the Mobile Crew throughout the entire workday. The Mobile Crew team travels by car from place to place providing services to paying customers. These customers hire TEACCH, which in turn, hires the individuals with ASD to work on the Mobile Crew. As with the One-to-One model, the job coach is available to assist clients with completing tasks, accommodate for fluctuating job performance, insure the accuracy and quality of completed work, and assist clients in the use of relaxation strategies.

The Mobile Crew model has the ability to accommodate each individual's needs. For example, the Job Coach can develop work schedules that take into account the length of day a person can work, and the number and length of breaks they need in order to complete the work without becoming frustrated or overwhelmed. The job coach has the option of assigning tasks based upon the strengths and interests of each member of the Mobile Crew. The biggest advantage of the Mobile Crew Model is providing training sites where the individual with ASD can develop or improve work skills for competitive employment, while at the same time earning a paycheck.

Group Shared Support Sites

For those individuals who have developed substantial work skills but still need on-going, intermittent support, there is the Group Shared Support Model. This model of supported employment consists of one job coach and between two and four persons with ASD who are employed directly by the company where they work. Typically, each individual with ASD who works at the Shared Support Site is hired to do a different job within the company. The individual must be able to complete most, if not all, aspects of his or her position with only intermittent support from a job coach. The TEACCH Supported Employment

Program has Shared Support Sites in bakeries, food services, grocery stores, warehouses, manufacturing, and laboratories.

People with ASD who work in this model benefit from having a job coach available on-site for either part or all of the work day. The job coaches typically split their time among the clients, focusing their attention on the person or situation needing it most at any one time.

Independent Placements

For individuals with the most independent work skills and minimal need for support, there is the Independent Model. This model consists of one job coach and 10 to 15 persons with ASD who work independently at their respective places of employment. The job coach travels from job site to job site providing support to individual clients and employers.

People with ASD in this model typically receive support from their job coach from 1 to 6 hours each week depending on the person's needs, the employer's needs, and the nature of the issues needing support. Support may increase or decrease within a given time period depending upon issues that arise. By providing the necessary amount of support each week, the job coach is able to minimize, or even prevent, problems through effective communication with the individual with ASD, the employers and supervisors, and co-workers. This 'long-term support' aspect of the Independent Model is a unique and effective aspect of TEACCH's Supported Employment program.

Assessment

Assessment is the cornerstone of successful employment. As others have noted (Smith et al., 1995), formal assessments utilizing standardized measures may not provide the most accurate information about an individual's vocational skills and potential in real-life settings. Informal, supplemental assessments that include direct observations across a variety of settings, coupled with interviews of the individual and knowledgeable others, provide more thorough and useful information. The assessment process itself needs to identify each individual's strengths and interests, not only the weaknesses. An individual's strengths and interests can provide a direction in the job search for individuals with ASD (LeBlanc, Schroeder, & Mayo, 1997). Further, Howlin (1997) noted that both Kanner and Asperger as well as current authors with ASD (e.g., Temple Grandin, Donna Williams) report that successful employment outcomes for adults with ASD are often based on their being able to use their special skill or interests.

Equally important during the assessment is determining each individual's unique characteristics of ASD and specific learning style, so that job coaches can develop teaching and support strategies that enable employees with ASD to use the skills they have on the job site. Thus, as described by Smith et al. (1995), the assessment needs to include the vocational and academic skills of the prospective employee as well as related skills and behaviors, communication skills, social skills, vocational behaviors, and coping skills. Most of the difficulties that individuals with ASD have at work are not due to lack of vocational skills. Rather, problems at work are typically related to communication difficulties, failure to follow social rules, the inability to work independently, obsessive behaviors, or resistance to changes in duties (Howlin, 1997). Other problem behaviors can relate to time factors or difficulty making judgments about the quality of work. Therefore, adaptations around these areas of functioning are often the most critical aspect of the job coach's responsibilities.

The Supported Employment assessment process includes an assessment of the fundamental characteristics of ASD. The social behaviors assessed include the individual's ability to work in proximity to others, to initiate and respond appropriately in social interactions, and to respond to multiple supervisors. Also, the ability to initiate and sustain appropriate behaviors during breaks has sometimes been the deciding factor in whether some clients can maintain a job. Communication skills that are most essential at work involve the ability to understand the directions or corrections of others, to initiate a request for help, or to notify someone when something is needed or when the job is complete. In addition, being able to communicate needing time off from work for any reason (e.g., sickness, doctor's appointment, or vacation) is important. The person's flexibility, ability to take on new tasks, and ability to control preoccupations during work time will also affect the type of jobs and work settings that are most appropriate.

As shown in Table 1, the assessment generally also includes a wide variety of specific vocational skills including, but not limited to, clerical skills, food preparation and domestic skills, gardening and landscaping, and basic skills related to stocking, packaging, sorting, assembly and disassembly activities. As the job coach assesses the individual's functioning in these activities, special attention is given to noting both the type and amount of visual support the individual needs to complete the task successfully and independently.

In addition to skill levels, behaviors that contribute to success in the work place are also assessed. For example, can the person move from area to area within a worksite without becoming distracted? Can the person arrange or provide transportation to and from a worksite? Sensory issues such as the individual's response to lighting, noises, and other potential distractions are other important observations. Further, it is important to observe noises or behaviors that the person with ASD exhibits that may have an impact on future co-workers. Additional vocational behaviors such as punctuality, time on task, stamina, distractibility, ability to make transitions, quality of work, rate of production, and ability to self monitor and correct mistakes will influence the type of jobs sought, the types of support provided, and the appropriate length of the work day. A more detailed account of the Supported Employment assessment process, the TEACCH Transition Assessment Profile (TTAP, a revision of the AAPEP), is in preparation.

Another important aspect of the assessment process is gathering information about the person's previous work history, such as whether the person has been employed before, what type of job(s) he or she has had, how long the job(s)

Table 11.1 Sample of Informal Supplemental Assessment Items for Employment

Clerical Skills	Library Skills
Typing	Using card catalogue
Data entry	Shelving books
Sorting (by letter and number)	Scanning shelves for books
Filing (folders and rolodex)	*Landscaping/Gardening Skills*
Photocopying	Weeding
Microfilming	Potting plants
Collating	Digging holes
Stapling	Mowing
Laminating	Using weed whacker
Stuffing envelopes	Trimming hedges
Using telephone book	Raking
Answering telephone	Planting/packaging seeds
Cutting paper	Picking vegetables
Shredding paper	*Food Service Skills*
Domestic Skills	Cutting, slicing, peeling foods
Dusting	Using stove and oven
Vacuuming	Using microwave
Sweeping	Loading dishwasher
Mopping	Scrubbing, washing pots
Wiping tables	Sorting and putting away clean dishes
Washing windows/mirrors	Filling condiment containers
Using washing machine	Serving food to others
Using dryer	Using cash register
Folding laundry	*Independent Functioning*
Sorting recycling	Arriving on time
Making bed	Returning from break on time
Warehouse/Stockroom Skills	Informing of schedule changes
Stocking and re-stocking	Organizing work materials
Scanning	Following daily schedule
Lifting	Following visual checklist, directions
Labeling/pricing	Following safety procedures
Vocational Characteristics	Prioritizing job responsibilities
Stamina (daily and weekly)	Personal hygiene, clothing
On-task time	Money management
Distractibility	Transportation skills
Transitions between tasks	
Mobility within tasks	
Sustained quality	
Sustained pace	
Correction of mistakes	

lasted, and the employee's, employer's, and family's perspectives on why the job(s) did not succeed. This information helps predict what behaviors or issues need to be addressed for future jobs to be successful, and it will also help in the construction of the individual's resume. Throughout the assessment process, sharing information with family members, caregivers, or others who know that person well will augment understanding of the client's needs and interests, thereby improving the chances of a successful placement.

An informal but thorough initial assessment typically takes approximately 60 hours, but has been known to range from 25 to 80 hours, depending on how well the individual's communication and social skills are already known and on how many vocational settings are assessed. Assessment is actually an on-going activity that continues after the individual has been placed in a job. A successful placement involves monitoring the individual's functioning and the job requirements, so that new skills can be taught, and the job restructured as needed.

Job Placements

To date, the SE program has placed individuals in jobs in the areas of office or clerical work, grocery stores, warehouses, laboratories, food service, janitorial work, landscaping, and libraries. See Table 2 for a listing of possible jobs in these areas. It should be noted that sometimes jobs that neurotypical employees dislike are actually appealing to individuals with ASD.

Office Jobs/Clerical Skills

Many successful clerical jobs for individuals with ASD take advantage of their strengths in attention to detail and desire to organize things into their proper places. Skills developed in school as simple sorting tasks (color, size, number, letter, etc.) can evolve into filing, mailing, cataloging, or shelving materials. Computer skills can lead to jobs in data processing, data entry, or bookkeeping. The interest in precision of many people with ASD makes many office jobs a good fit. However, office jobs that have a large social component or require flexibility, language processing, and judgment (such as answering the telephone or receptionist) can be much more challenging for individuals with ASD.

Grocery Jobs

Many community grocery stores are willing to hire individuals with limited work experience. We have had the greatest success in placements where the skills required match the strengths of the individuals. Stocking shelves, pricing merchandise, and scanning merchandise for inventories are tasks that lend themselves to the strengths of individuals with ASD and to the use of visual strategies. Although we have individuals who are successful as cashiers or baggers, these jobs are more challenging because of both the social elements and the increased time pressures involved in these positions.

Warehouse Jobs/Stocking Jobs

Packaging, labeling, inventory, and unpacking are all jobs that can build on the strengths of an individual with ASD. Problematic issues in these settings frequently involve how best to adapt large, noisy settings with lots of activity, in order to minimize over stimulation and maximize our clients' attention to their tasks.

Table 11.2   Examples of Supported Employment Jobs

Office Jobs	*Grocery Jobs*
Accountant	Bagging
Mail Room	Stocking
File Clerk	Pricing
Library	Cashier
Payroll	Scan Stock for Correct Pricing
Data Processing/Data Entry	Butcher
Microfilming	Produce Preparation
Bank	*Laboratory Jobs*
Office Assistant (Filing, Mailing, Typing)	Animal Handling
Stocking/Warehouse Jobs	Clerk Cage Washing
Inventory Clerk	Mix Food for Animals
Shipping and Receiving	Wash Glassware
Gift Basket Preparation	Sample Room Attendant
Pre-Label Supplies or Cartons	*Janitorial Jobs*
Order Packaging	Cleaning Crew
Retail Stores	Laundry Room
Quality Control	Food Service
Food Service Jobs	Warehouses
Line Server	Office Settings
Food Preparation	Grocery Stores
Dish/Pot Washer	Schools
Cashier	Retirement Homes
'Bus Boy'	Hotels
Dining Room Attendant	
Sort and Wrap Silverware	
Other Jobs	
Landscaping	
Animal Care	
Auto Repair	
Arts and Crafts	
Copy Machine Repair	
Truck Driver	

Laboratory Jobs

There are a number of jobs in research facilities that build on the visual strengths and interests of the individual with ASD without providing challenging social environments. Many laboratory jobs can be done in a setting removed from frequent social interruptions, and frequently the activities have great predictability and require someone who attends to details.

Food Service Jobs

Fast food restaurants are often not good settings for individuals with ASD because of the hectic work pace, the instability of the work force, the multiple job functions each worker must perform, and the crowded physical space. However, there are jobs in other food service facilities that may be appropriate. Large food service operations such as cafeterias in hospitals, retirement communities, university settings, big companies, or large other facilities generally allow for specialized job functions. Also, the longer timelines for the preparation of food or cleaning in these larger settings have a greater potential to meeting the tempo of the person with ASD.

Janitorial Jobs

Cleaning jobs have the advantage of building on skills that have generally been taught for years both at home and at school. However, these activities can be difficult because of the judgment involved in knowing whether something is clean or dirty. Visual systems developed for these settings emphasize helping the individual have a sequenced and organized approach to the tasks, and know when tasks are finished. An advantage of janitorial jobs is that the individual typical works in a setting removed from unpredictable social interactions.

Other Jobs

There are many other job possibilities for individuals with ASD based purely on the skills and interests of the person with ASD. Limiting factors usually relate to the social judgment and time demands of the job, not to the specific skills required.

Job Development

The job development process starts with the information that has been gathered from the client and family during the assessment process. In addition to obtaining information about the person's skills and behaviors, it is essential to determine both the client and family's needs and job expectations. For example, are there certain types of employment they will not consider? Are there financial issues that affect how much money the person needs to make? In interviewing clients about what work situations are most desirable and least desirable, it may be helpful to have them write down the five things they would prefer in a new job situation and the five things that they would like to avoid. Previous work experiences can help them in this process. Through these interviews with the client and family, the job coach can assist the client in the development of a resume and the job search.

The next step in the job development process is selecting potential work. It is important to look for work environments where there is stability in the work force and job requirements. Frequent changes in either personnel or job demands are not a good match for these individuals who need predictability in their activities. Job settings where the supervisors and co-workers are open to working with individuals with atypical behavior are essential. Sites where the productivity demands are steady and moderate are preferable to sites with fluctuating expectations or a high priority on speed.

To locate potential jobs, job coaches explore a variety typical resources such as newspapers/classified ads, temporary agencies, the internet, and personal contacts. As with the typical work force, personal contacts and employer referrals (where an employer of a person with ASD refers another employer to us) are often more successful.

The Supported Employment Program job coaches have found that they are more successful when they contact perspective employers face-to-face than when they attempt to make contact via the telephone. With the permission of the prospective job candidate, sharing information about the applicant's ASD is generally helpful. The facts that individuals with ASD will want to do the job the same way each day, that they don't spend a lot of time communicating and socializing about non-work topics, and that they are generally dedicated to their jobs and unwilling to miss work even when they are sick can all be significant advantages to an employer looking for a dedicated worker.

The participation of job applicants with ASD in the interview process varies according to their communication skills and preferences. We encourage more capable clients to practice job interviews in advance and to bring the job coach with them to the interview when company policies permit this. Often the job candidates need assistance in knowing how to dress and what to bring and not bring to the job interview. For some of our less verbally communicative clients, we try to arrange a job sampling session rather than an interview so they can demonstrate their skills to the prospective employer.

The job coaches also work with the clients to complete the job applications and to help to explain any 'red flags' in their work history that may be a source of concern to the employer.

Visual Structure

A unique aspect of the TEACCH SE Program is the use of visual strategies to increase the independence and job performance of the employees with ASD. As mentioned previously, the use of schedules, work/activity systems, and visual instructions has been shown to improve transitions, independence in following work lists, and the generalization of skills across settings, in addition to reducing inappropriate behaviors (Mesibov et al., 2002).

The physical structure of the work setting may need to be adjusted in order to provide clear visual and physical boundaries or to minimize distractions for the worker with ASD. In some settings, this can mean defining clear places for employees to go during their break times. For others, it may be rearranging their work spaces so as to direct their attention away from potential distractions or to minimize the chance for others to move into their work space.

The schedule (which essentially tells the person with ASD where to be) and the work/activity system (which specifically informs the person of what to do, how much to do, when he or she will be finished, and what next) may be combined into a single 'to do' list in a job setting. These systems utilize the type of visual cue that is most understandable to the individual with ASD (written directions, pictures, objects, etc.). In some settings, the job coach develops a template for each day's activities which includes the times to work, take a break, eat lunch, go home, etc., and leaves blanks for the supervisor to fill in the specific jobs of each day. When possible, these systems are blended in with the employer's natural systems of giving instructions in the work settings. In fact, a number of employers have found that the visual systems constructed by job coaches for the employees with ASD have also been helpful for their neurotypical co-workers.

A critical aspect of structure within the work setting is the use of visual instructions for completing specific jobs. These directions help the individual know how to do the job, what sequence of steps to follow, and/or when to stop. The job coach works to develop the most concrete and simple instructions that can be blended into the environment and made durable. The types of visual instructions vary greatly depending on the needs of the individual, the job, and the work setting. Some individuals will need visual instructions that tell them how to perform a task or diagrams the sequence of steps; examples include making labels with Dewey decimals for books of different sizes in a library, written step-by-step directions for sending out packages in a warehouse, and steps for cleaning a house. Picture directions can be jigs for assembling parts for a piece of manufacturing equipment, planting seeds in a greenhouse, or stacking dishes on a tray. For more concrete learning styles, a three-dimensional jig or 'cut-out' jig may help workers to measure the right amount of butter for baking, or to package the right number of seeds for planting.

For some jobs and workers, structure involves concrete organizational strategies that help to organize the materials and to limit the focus of attention. These strategies include using containers to organize work materials, such as providing buckets or baskets for cleaning supplies. Limiting the area one attends to can be accomplished in many ways. For example, in a landscaping job traffic cones can be used to indicate where to mow, or hoops can be used to show where to weed or mulch. Color-coding, highlighting, and labeling are other helpful strategies of drawing the person's attention to the relevant materials.

Communication Skills

Visual systems serve as a receptive communication aid by helping people with ASD to understand others' expectations. The expressive communication skills of the employee with ASD are also important for job success. Employees need to be able to let their supervisors know when they do not know what to do or do not understand a direction. They also need to know how to inform others when they are finished with a job, or if they run out of materials or have the wrong materials. Even more challenging is knowing how and when to make a sick leave or vacation request. Communication skills also affect relationships with co-workers.

The TEACCH approach to communication (see Chapter 6, Communication) is applicable to adults in Supported Employment situations. Assessing the workers' spontaneous communication within the work context allows the job coach to identify what system the individual uses to communicate (verbal, written, picture, etc.) and the content or function of the communication (requesting, sharing, information, etc.). Based on this assessment the job coach can help develop a communication system to address clients' needs in the work context.

A typical communication system at work involves a system for asking for help. For some individuals, all that is needed is a written reminder that says "if you need help, ask your supervisor." For others, the instructions may need to be more specific: "if you run out of materials or if something is broken ask _____." More concrete visual strategies may include having available a picture of the job coach or supervisor and pictures of the materials being used for a job. When additional materials are needed, the worker is taught to put the picture of what is needed next to the supervisor's or job coach's picture and then give this card to the supervisor or job coach. For individuals who do not know what to do when they finished a particular job, the job coach might develop a picture or written list of some jobs to do if they run out of work.

For more verbal individuals, telephone scripts may be developed for the individual to use when he or she is sick and needs to call and let the supervisor know. Similarly, written forms or verbal scripts are used as a means of requesting time off from work.

Social aspects of communication are also very important in maintaining a job. Job coaches work on teaching the workers with ASD to greet their co-workers appropriately. They also work with co-workers to let them know that a lack of greeting or problems with eye-contact are not intended as rudeness, but are part of ASD. Interacting with customers or with co-workers during breaks can be the most challenging issue of employment, and it can easily lead to the loss of a job. Social stories, social rules, and social scripts are all utilized to teach the person with ASD where, when, and with whom they may communicate. For the overly verbal employee, these measures are also utilized to teach them what topics to talk about and for how long they may talk. The schedule is often utilized as a concrete way of letting the individual with ASD know when they can talk about a repetitive topic. 'Question cards' can be used as tokens to indicate how many times during the day the worker can ask repetitive questions.

Social and Recreational Issues

The success of the TEACCH Supported Employment program is due in part to the fact that job performance and satisfaction are viewed as only part of the person's life. For a person to be successful on the job, other aspects of his or her life must be at least adequate. Job coaches must consider clients' living situations, with special emphasis on their social outlets and what they do for fun or recreation. Individuals with satisfactory (according to their own appraisal) social outlets and active recreational pursuits outside of work will be more satisfied focused and calm within the job.

Social groups (See Chapter 7, Social Skills) have been an important aspect of the Supported Employment program; groups have met several times a month, and most clients and job coaches have attended. These groups serve as a social outlet for the clients, and they also give the job coaches who are doing intermittent, long-term support an informal chance to check in with their clients to see how they are doing and to ask about issues on the job.

Program Evaluation

During the first 13 years of TEACCH's Supported Employment Program, 218 individuals were placed in 298 jobs in the community. As of January, 2002, the average hourly wage was $6.65 with a range of $5.15 to $16.66 with benefits. The average number of hours worked per week was 22.5 with a range of 4 to 56 hours.

During the period from 1997–2002, the retention rate at 6 months after placement was 89% and at 12 months after initial placement was 85%. These rates were even higher when events such as elimination of the work site, clients' moving out of the area, and clients' electing to take a different job were taken into account. When those situations were factored out, the retention rate was 96% at 6 months and 94% at 12 months.

SUMMARY

Assessment and treatment techniques originally developed in clinics and classrooms for children with ASD have successfully been extended to help adults with ASD maximize their ability to function independently in both residential and vocational settings. Through respect for the Culture of Autism, use of Structured Teaching techniques, and collaboration with families, other agencies, employers, and the broader community, the TEACCH program has enabled adults with ASD to engage in meaningful work and to have enjoyable personal lives.

REFERENCES

Allison, D.B., Basile, V.C., & MacDonald, R.B. (1991). Brief report: Comparative effects of antecedent exercise and lorazepam on the aggressive behavior of an autistic man. *Journal of Autism and Developmental Disorders, 21*, 89–94.

Anderson, M.D., Sherman, J.A., Sheldon, J.B., & McAdam, D. (1997). Picture activity schedules and engagement of adults with mental retardation in a group home. *Research in Developmental Disabilities, 18*, 231–250.

Ballaban-Gil, K., Rapin, I., Tuchman, R., & Shinnar, S. (1996). Longitudinal examination of the behavioral, language and social changes in a population of adolescents and young adults with autistic disorder. *Pediatric Neurology, 15*, 217–223.

Bambara, L.M. & Ager, C. (1992). Using self-scheduling to promote self directed leisure activity in home and community settings. *Journal of the Association for Persons with Severe Handicaps, 17,* 67–76.

Bondy, A.S. & Frost, L.A. (1994). The picture exchange communication system. *Focus on Autistic Behavior, 9,* 1–19.

Browder, D.M. & Minarovic, T. (2000). Utilizing sight words in self instruction training for employees with moderate mental retardation in competitive jobs. *Education and Training in Mental Retardation and Developmental Disabilities, 35,* 78–89.

Cautela, J.R. & Gorden, J. (1978). *Relaxation: A comprehensive manual for adults, children and children with special needs.* Champaign, Illinois: Research Press.

Clarke, S., Dunlap, G., & Vaughn, B. (1999). Family-centered assessment-based intervention to improve behavior during an early morning routine. *Journal of Positive Behavior Intervention, 1,* 235–241.

Community Services for Autistic Adults and Children (CSAAC). (1995). *Adults residential program. Adult vocational program* [Brochure]. Rockville, MD: Author.

Dooley, P., Wilczenski, F.L., & Torem, C. (2001). Using an activity schedule to smooth school transitions. *Journal of Positive Behavior Interventions, 3,* 57–61.

Dyer, K. (1989). The effects of preference on spontaneous verbal requests in individuals with autism. *Journal of the Association for Persons with Severe Handicaps, 14,* 184–189.

Dyer, K., Dunlap, G., & Winterling, V. (1990). The effects of choice-making on the serious problem behaviors of students with developmental disabilities. *Journal of Applied Behavior Analysis, 23,* 515–524.

Elliot, R.O., Dobbin, A.R., Gordon, D.R., & Soper, H.V. (1994). Vigorous exercise versus general motor training activities: Effects on maladaptive and stereotypic behaviors of adults with both autism and mental retardation. *Journal of Autism and Developmental Disorders, 24,* 565–576.

Elliot, R.O., Hall, K, & Soper, H. (1991). Analog language teaching versus natural language teaching: Generalization and retention of language learning for adults with autism and mental retardation. *Journal of Autism and Developmental Disorders, 21,* 433–448.

Everard, M.D. (1976, July). Mildly autistic young people and their problems. Paper presented at the International Symposium on Autism, St. Gallen, Switzerland.

Favell, J.E. & Cannon, P. (1976). Evaluation of entertainment materials for severely retarded persons. *American Journal of Mental Deficiency, 81,* 357–361.

Federal Register. (1984, September 25). *Developmental Disabilities Act of 1984.* Report 98-1074, Section 102 (11) (F).

Flannery, B. & Horner, R. (1994). The relationship between predictability and problem behavior for students with severe disabilities. *Journal of Behavioral Education, 4,* 157–176.

Giddan, J.J. & Giddan, N.S. (1993). *European farm communities for autism.* Toledo: Medical College of Ohio Press.

Goldberg, R.T., McClean, M.M., LaVigna, R., Fratolillo, J., & Sullivan, R.T. (1990). Transition of persons with developmental disability from sheltered employment to competitive employment. *Mental Retardation, 28,* 299–304.

Grandin, T. (1995). *Thinking in pictures: And other reports from my life with autism.* New York: Random House.

Hall, L.J., McClannahan, L., & Krantz, P.J. (1995). Promoting independence in integrated classrooms by teaching aides to use activity schedules and decreased prompts. *Education and Training in Mental Retardation and Developmental Disabilities, 30,* 208–217.

Holmes, D.L. (1990). Community-based services for children and adults with autism: The Eden family of programs. *Journal of Autism and Developmental Disorders, 20,* 339–351.

Holmes, D. (1997). *Autism through the lifespan: The Eden model.* Maryland: Woodbine House.

Howlin, P. (1997). *Autism: Preparing for adulthood.* London: Routledge.

Howlin, P., Goode, S., Hutton, J., & Rutter, M. (2004). Adult outcome for children with autism. *Journal of Child Psychology and Psychiatry, 45,* 212–229.

Juhrs, P.D. (1988). *Community Services for Autistic Adults and Children Vocational Program Overview.* Unpublished manuscript.

Kanner, L. & Eisenberg, L. (1956). Early infantile autism. *American Journal of Orthopsychiatry, 26,* 55–65.

Kanner, L., Rodriguez, A., & Ashenden, B. (1972). How far can autistic children go in matters of social adaptation? *Journal of Autism and Childhood Schizophrenia, 2,* 9–33.

Kay, B.R. (1990). Bittersweet Farms. *Journal of Autism and Developmental Disorders, 20,* 309–322.

Keel, J.H., Mesibov, G.B., & Woods, A.V. (1997). TEACCH Supported Employment Program, *Journal of Autism and Developmental Disorders, 27,* 3–10.

Krantz, P.J., MacDuff, M.T., & McClannahan, L.E. (1993). Programming participants in family activities for children with autism: Parents' use of photographic activity schedules. *Journal of Applied Behavior Analysis, 26,* 137–138.

Landesman, S. (1987). The changing structure and function of institutions: A search for optimal group care environments. In S. Landesman & P. Vietze (Eds.), *Living environments and mental retardation* (pp. 79–126). Washington, D.C.: American Association on Mental Retardation.

LaVigna, G.W. (1983). The Jay Nolen Center: A community-based program. In E. Schopler & G.B. Mesibov (Eds.), *Autism in adolescents and adults* (pp. 381–410). New York: Plenum Press.

LeBlanc, J.M., Schroeder, S. & Mayo, L. (1997). A life-span spproach in the education and treatment of persons with autism. In D.J. Cohen & F.R. Volkmar (Eds.) *Handbook of autism and pervasive developmental disorders* (pp. 934–946). New York: Wiley and Sons.

Lettick, A.L. (1983). Benhaven. In E. Schopler & G.B. Mesibov (Eds.), *Autism in adolescents and adults* (pp. 355–379). New York: Plenum Press.

Lockyer, L. & Rutter, M. (1969). A five to fifteen year follow-up study of infantile psychosis, III. Psychological aspects. *British Journal of Psychiatry, 115,* 865–882.

Lockyer, L. & Rutter, M. (1970). A five to fifteen year follow-up study of infantile psychosis: IV. Patterns of cognitive abilities. *British Journal of Social and Clinical Psychology, 9,* 152–163.

Lotter, V. (1974a). Factors related to outcome in autistic children. *Journal of Autism and Childhood Schizophrenia, 4,* 263–277.

Lotter, V. (1974b). Social adjustment and placement of autistic children in Middlesex: A follow-up study. *Journal of Autism and Childhood Schizophrenia, 4,* 11–32.

MacDuff, G.S., Krantz, P.J., & McClannahan, L.E. (1993). Teaching children with autism to use photographic activity schedules: maintenance and generalization—a complex response chain. *Journal of Applied Behavior Analysis, 26,* 89–97.

Mawhood, L. & Howlin, P. (1999). The outcome of a supported employment scheme for high-functioning adults with autism or Asperger syndrome. *Autism, 3,* 229–254.

McGee, G.G., Almeida, M.C., Sulzer-Azaroff, B., & Feldman, R.S. (1992). Promoting reciprocal interactions via peer incidental teaching. *Journal of Applied Behavioral Analysis, 25,* 117–126.

McGimsey, J.F. & Favell, J.E. (1988). The effects of increased physical exercise on disruptive behavior in retarded persons. *Journal of Autism and Developmental Disorders, 18,* 167–180.

Mesibov, G.B. (1983). Diagnosis and assessment of autistic adolescents and adults. In E. Schopler & G.B. Mesibov (Eds.), *Diagnosis and assessment in autism* (pp. 227–238). New York: Plenum Press.

Mesibov, G.B., Browder, D.M., & Kirkland, C. (2002). Using individualized schedules as a component of positive behavioral support for students with developmental disabilities. *Journal of Positive Behavior Interventions, 4,* 73–79.

Mesibov, G.B., Schopler, E., Schaffer, B., & Landrus, R. (1988). *Adolescent and Adult Psychoeducational Profile (AAPEP).* Austin, TX: Pro-Ed.

Mesibov, G.B., Schopler, E., Schaffer, B., & Michal, N. (1989). Use of the Childhood Autism Rating Scale with autistic adolescents and adults. *Journal of the American Academy of Childhood Adolescent Psychiatry, 28,* 538–541.

Mesibov, G.B. & Shea, V. (1980, March). *Social and interpersonal problems of autistic adolescents.* Paper presented at the meeting of the Southeastern Psychological Association, Washington, DC.

Mesibov, G.B., Troxler, M., & Boswell, S. (1988). Assessment in the classroom. In E. Schopler & G.B. Mesibov (Eds.), *Diagnosis and assessment in autism* (pp. 261–270). New York: Plenum Press.

Meyer, R.N. (2001). *Asperger Syndrome Employment Workbook*. London: Jessica Kingsley.

Parks, C. (2001). *Exiting Nirvana*. New York: Little, Brown and Company.

Pierce, K.L. & Schreibman, L. (1994). Teaching daily living skills to children with autism in unsupervised settings through pictorial self-management. *Journal of Applied Behavior Analysis, 27*, 471–481.

Quill, K. (1998). Environmental supports to enhance social-communication. *Seminars in Speech and Language, 19*, 407–422.

Rosenthal-Malek, A. & Mitchell, S. (1997). The effects of exercise on the self stimulatory behaviors and positive responding of adolescents with autism. *Journal of Autism and Developmental Disabilities, 27*, 193–202.

Rusch, F.R. & Mithaug, D.E. (1980). *Vocational training for mentally retarded adults: A behavior analytic approach*. Champaign, IL: Research Press.

Rutter, M. (1970). Autistic children: Infancy to adulthood. *Seminars in Psychiatry, 2*, 435–450.

Rutter, M., Greenfield, D., & Lockyer, L. (1967). A five to fifteen year follow-up study of infantile psychosis, II. *Social and behavioral outcome British Journal of Psychiatry, 113*, 1183–1199.

Rutter, M. & Lockyer, L. (1967). A five to fifteen year follow-up study of infantile psychosis: I Description of sample. *British Journal of Psychiatry, 113*, 1169–1182.

Schafer, M.S., Wehman, E., Kregel, J., & West, M. (1990). National supported employment initiative: A preliminary analysis. *American Journal of Mental Retardation, 95*, 316–327.

Schopler, E. & Mesibov, G.B. (1983). *Autism in adolescents and adults*. New York: Plenum Press.

Schopler, E., Mesibov, G.B., & Hearsey, K.A. (1995). Structured teaching in the TEACCH system. In E. Schopler & G.B. Mesibov (Eds.). *Learning and Cognition in Autism* (pp. 243–268). New York: Plenum Press.

Schopler, E., Mesibov, G.B., Shigley, R.H., & Bashford, A. (1984). Helping autistic children through their parents: The TEACCH model. In E. Schopler and G.B. Mesibov (Eds.), *The effects of autism on the family* (pp. 65–81). New York: Plenum Press.

Schopler, E., Reicher, R.J., DeVillis, R.F., & Daly, K. (1980). Toward objective classification of childhood autism: Childhood Autism Rating Scale (CARS). *Journal of Autism and Developmental Disorders, 10*, 91–103.

Schopler, E., Reichler, R.J., & Renner, B.R. (1988). *The Childhood Autism Rating Scale (CARS)*. Los Angeles: Western Psychological Services.

Simonson, L.R., Simonson, S.M., & Volkmar, F.R. (1990). Benhaven's residential program. *Journal of Autism and Developmental Disorders, 20*, 323–338.

Smith, M., Belcher, R., & Juhrs, P. (1995). *A guide to successful employment for individuals with autism*. Baltimore, MD: Brookes.

Smith, M.D. & Coleman, E. (1986). Managing the behavior of adults with autism in the job setting. *Journal of Autism and Developmental Disorders, 16*, 145–154.

Sowers, J., Thompson, L.E., & Connis, R.T. (1979). The food service vocational training program: A model for training and placement of the mentally retarded. In G.T. Bellamy, G. O'Connor, & O.C. Karan (Eds.), *Vocational rehabilitation of severely handicapped persons* (pp. 181–205). Baltimore: University Park Press.

Van Bourgondien, M.E. & Elgar, S. (1990). The relationship between existing residential services and the needs of autistic adults. *Journal of Autism and Developmental Disorders, 20*, 299–308.

Van Bourgondien, M.E., Mesibov, G.B., & Castelloe, P. (1989, July). *Adaptation of clients with autism to group homes settings*. Paper presented at the national conference of the Autism Society of America, Seattle, WA.

Van Bourgondien, M.E. & Reichle, N.C. (1996). *The Carolina Living and Learning Center: An example of the TEACCH approach to residential and vocational training for adults with autism*. In G. Kristoffersen & E. Kristoffersen (Eds.), Status Pa Garden (pp. 155–169). Copenhagen: Parentes.

Van Bourgondien. M.E. & Reichle, N.C. (1997). *Residential treatment for individuals with autism*. In D.J. Cohen & F.R. Volkmar (Eds.), *Handbook of autism and pervasive developmental disorders* (pp. 691–706). New York: John Wiley and Sons.

Van Bourgondien, M.E. & Reichle, N.C. (2001). Evaluating treatment effects for adolescents and adults with autism in residential treatment settings. In E. Schopler, N. Yirmiya, C. Shulman, &

L.M. Marcus (Eds.), *Research basis for autism intervention* (pp. 187–197). New York: Kluwer Academic/Plenum Press.

Van Bourgondien, M.E., Reichle, N.C., & Schopler, E. (2003). Effects of a model treatment approach on adults with autism. *Journal of Autism and Developmental Disorders, 33*, 131–140.

Van Bourgondien, M.E. & Schopler, E. (1990). Critical issues in the residential care of people with autism. *Journal of Autism and Developmental Disorders, 20*, 391–400.

Van Bourgondien, M.E. & Schopler, E. (1996). Intervention for adults with autism. *Journal of Rehabilitation, 62*, 65–71.

Van Bourgondien, M. E. & Woods, A. V. (1992). Vocational possibilities for high-functioning adults with autism. In E. Schopler & G.B. Mesibov (Eds.) *High-functioning individuals with autism* (pp. 227–239). New York: Plenum Press.

Wall, A.J. (1990). Group homes in North Carolina for children and adults with autism. *Journal of Autism and Developmental Disabilities, 20*, 353–366.

Watson, L.R., Lord, C., Schaffer, B., & Schopler, E. (1989). *Teaching spontaneous communication to autistic and developmentally handicapped children.* Austin, TX: Pro-Ed.

Wehman, P. (1981). *Competitive employment: New horizons for severely disabled individuals.* Baltimore: Paul Brookes.

Wehman, P., Hill, M., Hill, J.M., Brooke, V., Pendleton, P., & Britt, C. (1985). Competitive employment for persons with mental retardation: A follow up 6 years later. *Mental Retardation, 23*, 274–281.

Williams, D. (1992). *Nobody Nowhere.* London: Corgi Books.

CHAPTER 12

Training Issues

INTRODUCTION

Programmatic efforts of TEACCH and other comprehensive service programs for people with autism spectrum disorders (ASD) target not only the clients themselves, but also those who work with them. Indeed, these initiatives have broadened our identification of the client to include not just the person with ASD, but also his or her parents, teachers, peers, residential program staff, employer, etc. The setting for intervention has changed from the insulated clinic office to the entire community. Every day, people with ASD interact with others who may know little or nothing about ASD. In the absence of special instruction about ASD, some community members may have a narrow or stereotyped view of the disorder learned from movies, sensationalized media accounts, or popular books. Indeed, much of the information about ASD that reaches the general public is vague or outdated at best, and misleading or erroneous at worst. One job of service programs to teach the general public about this perplexing disorder and its implications for social, personal, and educational functioning. This information is particularly needed by those who have little formal training in psychology, special education, or child development. However, even people with professional training, who are more familiar with ASD, need to be kept abreast of new developments in the field. This chapter will describe issues and TEACCH practices in inservice training for the many different types of professional staff members who come into contact with people with ASD.

TEACHER TRAINING PROGRAMS

Overview

Our understanding of how to educate students with ASD is constantly changing as a result of research and program evaluation. An experienced teacher who was originally trained more than 30 years ago would have been taught that parents cause ASD in their children, and that to help children with ASD we must remove them from their homes (Bettelheim, 1967). Even teachers trained more recently may have learned that students with ASD are 'untestable.' Furthermore, the recent proliferation of the diagnosis of Asperger Syndrome has left many special education and regular education teachers confused about educational goals and techniques for these students. There is a need for teacher training programs that can provide teachers with the most current and useful knowledge in the field. Because rigorous program evaluation studies and clear descriptions of successful training programs are scarce, there is disagreement in the professional literature as to how to deliver inservice training. This chapter will present key issues in the field of teacher training, with an emphasis on the elements of training that are necessary to create changes in the classroom. One model of teacher training procedures implemented by TEACCH will be described at the end of the chapter.

General Issues

Goals

The first step in developing a teacher training program is identifying its desired outcomes. Indirectly, all programs intend to improve the education of students with ASD. The challenge lies in determining what has to happen to teachers in order to reach this goal. Trainers should have a clear idea of their desired outcome, and should design their training program with that outcome in mind. One basic goal is to achieve trainee satisfaction with the intervention program. However, this should not be the only goal of a training program; rather, it is seen as a prerequisite for trainee motivation and ability to learn and implement new skills. Another necessary outcome, but again not a sufficient one, is increased factual knowledge. Related to new knowledge is a change in attitudes and beliefs. Some training programs present a new way of thinking about ASD, or new ways of interpreting the behavior of people with ASD. For example, the TEACCH program and others train teachers to identify the underlying function of problem behaviors, rather than teaching them traditional contingency-based behavior modification strategies (Anderson, Albin, Mesaros, Dunlap, & Morelli-Robbins, 1993; Schopler, Mesibov, & Hearsey, 1995). If training can change the attitudes of trainees, it may go a step further and change the philosophy of schools or intervention programs (Fredericks & Templeman, 1990). This is another potential outcome, although a rather ambitious one.

Many programs strive to teach new, practical skills. For instance, Dyer, Williams, and Luce (1991) described a program that trained teachers to use naturalistic communication strategies. Acquisition of new skills is an outcome that is easy to measure: Can teachers use the skills or not? Several experts, however, have argued that a much more important question is: "Do teachers use the skills at school once training is over?" (Joyce & Showers, 1995; Whelan & Simpson, 1996). The few program evaluators who have asked this question have found disappointing results. Based on her knowledge of the literature and her own experience with training teachers, Showers (1990) asserted that those researchers who make the effort to investigate often find that skill-based training programs result in absolutely no implementation once teachers return to their classrooms. She has noticed that even if teachers enthusiastically practice the skills during training, transfer of training to the classroom is not automatic. Because of this phenomenon, it is clear that the overarching goals of training programs should be implementation and maintenance. Unless these goals are met, the impact of any training program on students in classrooms will be limited.

Cost-Benefit Analysis

Considering the low rate of implementation of learned techniques, it is wise to conduct a cost-benefit analysis when designing a training program. Trainers must ask themselves whether the amount of change they can create in classrooms is worth the cost in time and resources. Training programs can be very expensive, and schools must be informed consumers. Fees for training programs can include rental of a training site, payment of trainers and support staff, materials, and refreshments, not to mention travel and lodging if trainees travel far from home. If trainees must take time away from work, the cost of substitute teachers is added. Such factors as the duration of the program, its distance from trainees' work sites, the number of trainees trained at once, and the salary level of the trainers can also affect the cost of training. Costly programs must result in adequate implementation in order to be worthwhile. Thus, another important goal for training is to achieve an acceptable cost-benefit ratio. This puts the pressure on programs to deliver measurable results.

Location

There are equally convincing arguments for having training off-site and on-site. The answer for an individual program depends on its needs. Locating the program at the same school as the trainees minimizes their time off-work; it also eliminates travel time and costs. Programs that teach very specific skills could argue that on-site training would increase implementation. Trainers could directly observe any workplace characteristics, such as the size of classrooms, material resources, or teacher-student ratios which would affect application of new skills. For instance, teaching techniques that require one-on-one interaction with students would necessitate a high teacher-student ratio or a well-organized classroom that could accommodate some students working independently while others work with the teacher. Trainers who understand these workplace characteristics can keep them in mind while conducting training. Another advantage of on-site training is that it may be more convenient for some trainees. If training is incorporated into the regular work schedule, it does not conflict with other obligations. Also, teachers may be hesitant to schedule training during their free time.

On the other hand, conducting training off-site can eliminate distractions. The training is completely separate from teachers' everyday activities, and thus they can devote their full attention to it. Furthermore, off-site training is often more practical than on-site training. Trainees from several different schools, and perhaps several different states, can attend. It may be more cost-effective to train larger groups of teachers, perhaps even lowering the cost to the schools. And, trainees may place increased value on training for which they traveled some distance. If they and their schools are exerting much effort to receive training, they may exert more effort to ensure that the training pays off. An additional advantage of off-site training is that large groups of trainees can be divided into smaller groups who work together on hands-on activities. This provides practice with working in teams and creates the kind of collaborative atmosphere for which many schools strive.

Duration

The cost-benefit issue often drives decisions about how long training will last. Programs must impart as much information as possible to teachers without keeping them away from their students for too long. Schools may be unwilling to implement a highly effective training program if it is too costly and takes too much time. However, programs that establish longitudinal contact with schools seem to result in more implementation than short-term programs (Reichle et al., 1996). Anderson et al. (1993) suggested starting training with sessions which are close together in time, and then spreading later sessions out in order to allow teachers increased independence.

Who Should be Trained?

One would assume that training is intended for teachers of students with ASD. However, training may have more impact if it is aimed not just at individual teachers, but also at other school employees who have contact with the person with ASD or who can provide support to teachers (Anderson et al., 1993). Educational programs can be designed to be appropriate for principals, speech and language therapists, occupational therapists, psychologists, after-school staff, and other teachers who have contact with the student with ASD. In this way, teachers could have a network of colleagues to help them apply newly learned techniques, solve problems, and evaluate their implementation of techniques. Furthermore, if the training presents more general material, other school personnel could apply the techniques to their own areas of expertise. Joyce and Showers (1995) suggested creating a system of school personnel who provide each other with social support and coaching in applying and maintaining new skills.

For some training programs, the age of teachers is thought to have an effect on implementation. Interestingly, there is disagreement as to whether it is younger or older teachers who are less likely to implement new skills. Favell,

Favell, Riddle, and Risley (1984) asserted that it is not always cost-effective to train younger teachers, as they are more likely than older teachers to leave the profession soon after training. Conversely, Langone, Koorland, and Oseroff (1987) argued that older teachers may have been using the same teaching methods for a long time, and thus be less interested in learning new skills. On the other hand, older teachers may have the greatest need for current information about ASD. As a group they are further away from their pre-service training, and thus most likely to have outdated ideas.

It may be teacher attitudes, rather than age, that affect openness to change. Joyce and Showers (1988) interviewed the teachers they trained at one school to assess their involvement in activities that led to personal growth. Examples of these activities were professional workshops, going to plays, pursuing hobbies, having professional discussions with other teachers, and becoming involved in mentoring relationships. They divided the teachers into four 'states of growth,' identified by teachers' willingness to seek opportunities for growth: so-called gourmet omnivores, active consumers, passive consumers, and reticents. These four types existed on a continuum, with gourmet omnivores independently seeking out staff development opportunities, such as workshops and lectures, while teachers in the middle of the continuum willingly participated in growth opportunities, but only in those which they are required to attend. Reticents were unlikely to attend or benefit from growth opportunities. The majority (70%) of the teachers Joyce and Showers studied were passive consumers. These teachers tended to follow what their peers were doing, not seeking out opportunities on their own or engaging in activities that were not required. Although passive consumers were generally cooperative and attentive at required activities, they were unlikely to implement any skills they learn. This finding highlights the importance of identifying ways to ensure that all trainees will implement new skills.

Trainers-of-Trainers

Many training programs train future trainers at the same time they train teachers (Anderson et al., 1993; Peck, Killen, & Baumgart, 1989). This is cost-effective, in that it eliminates the need for separate training programs. Also, future trainers learn in a naturalistic setting. The relationship between current and future trainers is that of apprenticeship. Future trainers learn by observing trainers in action, and gradually assume some training responsibilities under close supervision.

Methods of Delivery

With the aforementioned general issues in mind, trainers face the difficult task of finding the optimal mode of delivery for their programs. Matching training methods to available facilities and schedules of trainees is essential because no one method alone is sufficient to meet most training goals. A combination of methods is more likely to accommodate the preferred learning styles of many different trainees. It also allows trainers to convey the same information in multiple ways without being repetitive.

Lectures

Lectures given by experts in the field, administrators, or experienced teachers are an efficient way to convey large amounts of information to large groups in a short period of time. Inservice lectures and accompanying handouts often provide teachers with the theory behind the new techniques they are learning, and may also present relevant research data. However, there is some controversy as to whether or not teachers' time should be spent learning theory. Some argue that teachers do not use the theory they learn, but rather prefer learning more practical information and skills (Schumm & Vaughn, 1995; Smith & Smith, 1985). Certainly, teachers appreciate learning concrete techniques that are easily implemented. However, concrete techniques may be difficult for teachers to adapt to novel situations. With an understanding of a program's philosophy and theories, teachers are ready for any potential application of the theories, and can feel more comfortable being creative with the program's components. Because of the diversity within the population of individuals with ASD, teachers continually face the challenge of how to deal with a behavior they may never have observed in another student.

Manuals

Written instructions and manuals can be useful because they allow trainees to learn material at their own pace. Manuals are also permanent, making it possible for teachers to review them when needed. A training program that consists solely of a manual is less expensive, as it eliminates the need for a trainer or travel to a training site. However, using a manual alone is insufficient because trainees are unable to ask questions or prove their comprehension of techniques. Furthermore, a manual cannot provide in-vivo practice, interactive feedback, or coaching, which are useful training methods to be discussed later in the chapter.

Demonstration

Demonstrations are a valuable teaching method that is left out of lecture-only training programs. Video or in-vivo demonstrations do not depend on trainees' academic skills, and are more interesting and informative to many trainees than lectures. Watching an effective trainer is an excellent way to translate theoretical material into practical techniques. When demonstrations are in-vivo with students with ASD, trainees can watch trainers adapt the skills to specific and novel situations. Researchers agree that it is optimal to implement demonstrations which very closely approximate real-life practice (Joyce & Showers, 1995). Some programs even conduct demonstrations in the actual settings and with the same students the trainees will be expected to teach (Anderson et al., 1993; Reid, Parsons, & Green, 1989).

Practice

Mohlman, Kierstead, and Gundlach (1982) identified three common barriers to teacher implementation of training techniques: a) not believing in the program's philosophy, b) thinking change will cost too much or require too much effort, and c) inability to apply theory to practical situations. All three of these barriers are more likely to be overcome if programs incorporate a practicum component. In this way, trainees can test out new techniques for themselves, getting direct proof of the program's efficacy, determining how costly and difficult implementation would be, and generating their own practical applications under a trainer's supervision. Researchers are beginning to insist that practicum components are essential to teacher training programs. Lectures, manuals, and demonstrations require only passive receipt of training. Allowing trainees to practice what they have learned from other methods makes them more active learners.

Training programs have developed several creative ways of allowing teachers to practice skills. They vary in their approximation of real school situations, and therefore in their cost. The method which is most removed from real life is applying skills hypothetically or through written case studies. Sigafoos, Kerr, Roberts, and Couzens (1994) taught new skills to teachers through lectures and handouts, and then had the teachers generate ways to apply the new skills to their own students. Trainers evaluated and added to the trainees' ideas. Other programs have used role play techniques, having other trainees act as students (Joyce & Showers, 1995). These trainees reported that acting as a student was helpful for them, as well as for the other trainees. Presumably, taking the student's perspective provided a clearer understanding of the methods, and also fostered greater empathy for students. Adams, Tallon, and Rimell (1980) examined the implementation of positive reinforcement techniques in a mental retardation facility after a one-week training program. They compared two training formats: lecture and role play. Trainees who learned the techniques in lecture format showed a sharp increase in positive reinforcement directly after training, but soon showed a steady decline. Trainees who practiced the techniques through role play also showed an increase after training, but then continued with a steady increase in their use of positive reinforcement.

If the above ways of practicing new skills can be effective, then a closer approximation of real-life practice should be even more useful. Some programs have teachers practice new techniques with their own students (Peck et al., 1989). Jones, Bender, and McLaughlin (1992) had trainees develop single-subject research projects to assess the efficacy of their program while learning it. The ultimate goal of their training program was to reduce special education referrals by proving to teachers that they could manage their own students' behavior. They started with lectures on behavioral techniques such as positive reinforcement and contingency plans. For the practicum component of their program, they taught teachers to collect data on one student's target behavior. For example, one teacher reduced a student's disruptive talking by making free time contingent on staying quiet in class. The teachers met regularly as a group to address problems in data collection, generate intervention techniques, and assess each other's progress in applying the techniques at school. At the end of the program, twelve of the 16 projects were successful in changing students' target behaviors.

There are many advantages of practice. Practice working with a student with ASD is much more informative than working with person pretending to have ASD. Practicing new skills can raise questions that may not be stimulated by lectures. Also, trainers are able to monitor trainees' acquisition of skills by observing them practice, and thus can determine which skills and which trainees need review or clarification. Another advantage of practice is that trainees can prove to their trainers and themselves that they have actually acquired the new skills. Non-practice methods allow trainees to prove that they have acquired knowledge, not skills. Schumm and Vaughn (1995) emphasize that trainees are more likely to implement new skills if they have already used them in practice.

Increasing Implementation and Maintenance

After devoting substantial time in training, trainers and trainees alike assume that change will occur in the classroom starting directly afterwards. Most of the time it does. But what about the following school year, when the teacher has a new group of students? What happens five years after training? What happens on a bad day, when no one is observing the teacher? Unfortunately, most of these questions remain unanswered because these studies have not been attempted—but the importance of ensuring implementation and maintenance cannot be overestimated. Training programs should include mechanisms for increasing implementation and maintenance, rather than simply assuming that since trainees enjoyed the program they will use the skills.

Design of follow-up methods is typically based on speculation as to why teachers fail to implement skills once they return to their classrooms. Assuming that the original training program was not faulty, and that teachers learned the skills and believed in the philosophy of the program, problems in implementation must relate to the school setting. On returning to school after training, teachers may face administrators who will not allocate resources for the new teaching techniques. Or, the teacher may feel isolated, no longer having fellow trainees with whom to discuss the techniques and solve problems. Teachers may have difficulty applying their new skills to individual students who are different from the students with whom they practiced in training. Relatedly, when teachers encounter a student with whom the techniques are not immediately effective, they may prematurely reject the new techniques as inadequate for their needs. Although a thorough practicum component or on-site training can help with many of these concerns, follow-up contact is a highly effective supplement or substitute.

Follow-up and Evaluation

Programs that include a follow-up component usually allow trainees several weeks of independence directly after training. Henney and Strong (1993) prescribed at least a five-day initial training period with two or more follow-up sessions. In their study comparing a school with this training schedule to a school with a shorter initial training period and more follow-up sessions, they discovered that the longer initial training resulted in greater knowledge of training techniques. Although Henney and Strong measured technique application, they unfortunately did not report results on this variable. Presumably, trainees need a strong knowledge base before they attempt to apply new techniques. Most programs that use follow-up techniques expect teachers to begin implementing the skills in their own classrooms directly after the initial training. Teachers can later return to the training setting to receive follow-up consultation, or trainers can visit trainees' classrooms to provide direct feedback. However this is done, the follow-up phase is a time for troubleshooting and refinement of skills. Also, any parts of training that are not being implemented can be reviewed and modified to fit the individual trainee's needs.

Smith and Smith (1985) reported that their follow-up component was very effective. Their claims must be viewed with caution, however, because their report described what they believed led to their program's success, rather than the results of rigorous research supporting their assertions. Although they identified implementation as the goal of their program, they gave no information about how this variable was operationalized and measured, nor did they report statistical analyses. After formal training, Smith and Smith had trainers supervise guided practice with the trainees' own students. They asserted that without this practice, there was only a two-percent implementation of the program. Peck et al. (1989) described a small-scale research study on the follow-up of their training program, using an across-subjects multiple baseline design. They had three teachers videotape their own classrooms, and then each teacher later reviewed the videotapes with the trainer. Rather than providing suggestions, the trainer's role was to encourage the teacher to devise new techniques to intervene with one student's target behavior. This method increased teacher implementation and decreased the students' target behaviors, but so did the more cost-effective alternative of having teachers describe their implementation verbally, without a video.

Some trainers address teachers' discomfort with direct feedback on their performance, because of concern that teachers' dislike of evaluation will lead them to avoid training programs that use follow-up, or that it will cause reactivity problems. That is, in order to avoid negative feedback teachers may act differently when they know they are being evaluated than they do without evaluation.

Coaching

Joyce and Showers (1995) proposed another answer to the evaluation problem. They developed a follow-up system called coaching. After the initial training, trainers evaluate and assist teachers' implementation of skills in their own classrooms. Once implementation improves, the trainer leaves the school setting and trainees become peer coaches. The goal of coaching is not evaluation, but rather for trainees to observe one another implementing techniques, and to share ideas. Joyce and Showers indicated that this system worked just as well as a traditional evaluation program. It also eliminated the necessity of training teachers to evaluate each other and the cost of trainers' time. Furthermore, coaching facilitated an atmosphere of collaboration. Joyce and Showers (1988) reported that an unpublished dissertation which presented a meta-analysis of training program components demonstrated that the highest effect size came from a combination of lecture, demonstration, practice, feedback, and in-class coaching. This effect size was 1.68, and the effect measured as an outcome was skill implementation. The effect size for a program using either lecture only or demonstration only was 0.5.

TEACCH SUMMER TRAINING PROGRAM

Program Description

TEACCH conducts its summer training in facilities large enough for a lecture hall and a spacious model classroom. Teachers come from within North Carolina, from other states, and even from other countries. The training consists of an intensive one-week (40 hours) summer course that combines theoretical information and practical applications, giving them equal emphasis. During each of eight one-week training sessions, 25 teachers are trained. Then, North Carolina teachers can receive on-site consultation from TEACCH therapists who can monitor their implementation of the techniques and help them troubleshoot and individualize the new skills. They may also attend a February inservice conference for two days of lectures and demonstrations on practical topics.

About one-half of the trainees at TEACCH summer training are teachers; a significant number of parents, administrators, psychologists, speech and language therapists, and occupational therapists also attend. TEACCH also includes 'shadow trainers' in its training program, who follow the trainers and learn by observing. Shadow trainers attend trainer meetings and are present for all training activities, sometimes taking the role of a trainer under the trainer's supervision. The shadow trainers have already served as trainees in the past, and are ready to be trainers after the shadow training experience is complete.

The format of TEACCH summer training is a combination of lectures, manuals, demonstrations, practice, feedback, and follow-up. The first day consists of lectures, while the following four days are dividing among lectures, work in a classroom, and small group work. The lectures are given by clinicians, experienced teachers, and psychoeducational therapists from TEACCH centers, who together provide participants with multiple perspectives on TEACCH methods, their theoretical basis, and implementation. The lectures cover topics central to the program's philosophy: characteristics of autism spectrum disorders, assessment, Structured Teaching, managing behavior, communication, independence and vocational training, and social and leisure skills (Schopler, 1989). Theory is a crucial component of the program because we assume that teachers need to understand the rationale behind the TEACCH methods in order to learn them fully and use them flexibly. A firm grasp of theory and rationale is more likely to lead to a true understanding of the techniques, which in turn can bolster motivation to use them once training is over. TEACCH training includes a packet of materials that supplement and reinforce the other aspects of the program. In this way, many of the benefits of manuals are obtained without while the limitations of a manual-only program are avoided.

The program also combines demonstrations with other important aspects of training, such as trainee practice. This practical component of TEACCH training is often viewed as the most important part of the program. Many teachers report that it is also the most enjoyable. Roughly one-third to one-half of a trainee's time is spent practicing techniques in a model classroom. The students are five youngsters who represent varying levels of functioning; teachers work with a different student each of the four days they spend in the model classroom. These youngsters are not the teachers' own students. This is seen as an advantage, because it aids in generalization. Teachers learn to apply TEACCH techniques to four very different students, and then return to their own schools and apply them to their own students. This method fosters the ability to generalize techniques to an ever-changing student population, which is required of teachers in the long run.

Trainees are organized into teams of four or five, and each team works with one student per day in the classroom. The trainee groups stay the same throughout the week, but they work with a different student and a different TEACCH trainer each day. Over the course of the week, each trainee rotates through specific roles: teacher, recorder, family liaison, communicator, or group organizer. Each segment of the practicum is organized as a problem-solving exercise. The trainer describes a problem to the team, the team collaborates to design a task that will address the problem, implements the task with the student, observes the student's response, receives feedback from the trainer to modify the task, and then implements the revised task with the child. At the end of this process there is an hour-long feedback session for the team, in which they discuss their experiences and observations with the trainer in the small group.

TEACCH also provides follow-up consultation for North Carolina teachers on request. Consultants visit trainees' classrooms and observe their implementation of skills, giving feedback as necessary. This is seen as an opportunity to individualize training more than was possible in the larger groups of the original training period. Also, consultation helps teachers to be more creative in applying the new skills to their own students. As for teachers' discomfort with receiving feedback on their performance, consultants minimize the focus on this purpose of follow-up. Rather, the more important goal is for teachers to use the consultants' greater experience to troubleshoot and reinforce the original training.

Research Findings

The effectiveness of TEACCH summer training programs was the subject of a master's thesis and a doctoral dissertation at the University of North Carolina—Chapel Hill (Grindstaff, 1998, 2000). In a sample of 101 participants who completed a week of summer training and returned survey data, knowledge of TEACCH principles and methodology increased significantly compared to their pre-training knowledge and compared to a control group, and was maintained 6 weeks later (N = 96 at follow-up). Further, trainees' use of Structured Teaching principles, in response to written case scenarios, increased significantly compared to their pre-training levels and compared to controls.

CONCLUDING COMMENTS

Given the variety of program components and trainee needs, there is not a standard prescription for the perfect training program. More rigorous program evaluation studies to help in determining which training components yield the highest levels of implementation and long-term maintenance are urgently needed. However, even if we did know exactly what sort of training program is the most effective in terms of these variables, there are additional important factors to consider. Schools must choose programs that fit with their resources and workplace characteristics. It is clear that schools must investigate programs thoroughly before choosing one. The strongest conclusion that can be drawn from the current research is that schools should select programs that create visible changes in the classrooms. In this way, teacher training can reach its intended target: the students.

REFERENCES

Adams, G.L., Tallon, R.J., & Rimell, P. (1980). A comparison of lecture versus role-playing in the training of the use of positive reinforcement. *Journal of Organizational Behavior Management, 2*, 205–212.
Anderson, J.L., Albin, R.W., Mesaros, R.A., Dunlap, G., & Morelli-Robbins, M. (1993). Issues in providing training to achieve comprehensive behavioral support. In J. Reichle & D.P. Wacker (Eds.), *Communication and Language Intervention Series: Vol. 3. Communicative alternatives to challenging behavior: Integrating functional assessment and intervention strategies* (pp. 363–396). Baltimore: Paul H. Brookes.
Bettelheim, B. (1967). *The empty fortress.* New York: Free Press.

Dyer, K., Williams, L., & Luce, S.C. (1991). Training teachers to use naturalistic communication strategies in classrooms for students with autism and other severe handicaps. *Language, Speech, and Hearing Services in Schools, 22*, 313–321.

Favell, J.E., Favell, J.E., Riddle, J.I., & Risley, T.R. (1984). Promoting change in mental retardation facilities: Getting services from the paper to the people. In W. P. Christian, G. T. Hannah & T. J. Glahn (Eds.), *Programming effective human services: Strategies for institutional change and client transition* (pp. 15–37). New York: Plenum.

Fredericks, H.D.B. & Templeman, T.P. (1990). A generic in-service training model. In: A. P. Kaiser & C. M. McWhorter (Eds.), *Preparing personnel to work with persons with severe disabilities* (pp. 301–317). Baltimore: Paul H. Brookes.

Grindstaff, J.P. (1998). *Attributions and autism: An evaluation of TEACCH's experiential training programs.* Unpublished master's thesis, University of North Carolina-Chapel Hill, Chapel Hill.

Grindstaff, J.P. (2000). Further evaluation of TEACCH's experiential training programs: Change in participants' knowledge, attributions, and use of structure. (Doctoral dissertation, University of North Carolina-Chapel Hill, 2000). Dissertation Abstracts International-B, 62, 5374.

Henney, M. & Strong, M. (1993). Two continuing education models for preparing teachers to use whole language. *Psychological Reports, 73*(3, Pt. 1), 745–746.

Jones, K.H., Bender, W.N., & McLaughlin, P. (1992). Implementation of Project RIDE: Responding to individual differences in education. *Journal of Instructional Psychology, 19*, 107–112.

Joyce, B. & Showers, B. (1988). *Student achievement through staff development.* New York: Longman.

Joyce, B. & Showers, B. (1995). *Student achievement through staff development: Fundamentals of school renewal* (2nd ed.). White Plains, NY: Longman.

Langone, J., Koorland, M., & Oseroff, A. (1987). Producing changes in the instructional behavior of teachers of the mentally handicapped through inservice education. *Education and Treatment of Children, 10*, 146–164.

Mohlman, G.G., Kierstead, J., & Gundlach, M. (1982). A research-based inservice model for secondary teachers. *Educational Leadership, 40*, 16–19.

Peck, C.A., Killen, C.C., & Baumgart, D. (1989). Increasing implementation of special education instruction in mainstream preschools: Direct and generalized effects of nondirective consultation. *Journal of Applied Behavior Analysis, 22*, 197–210.

Reichle, J., McEvoy, M., Davis, C., Rogers, E., Feeley, K., Johnston, S. et al. (1996). Coordinating preservice and in-service training of early interventionists to serve preschoolers who engage in challenging behavior. In L.K. Koegel, R.L. Koegel, & G. Dunlap (Eds.), *Positive behavioral support: Including people with difficult behavior in the community* (pp. 227–264). Baltimore: Paul H. Brookes.

Reid, D.H., Parsons, M.B., & Green, C.W. (1989). *Staff management in human services: Behavioral research and application.* Springfield, IL: Charles C. Thomas.

Schopler, E. (1989). Principles for directing both educational treatment and research. In C. Gillberg (Ed.), *Diagnosis and treatment of autism* (pp. 167–183). New York: Plenum.

Schopler, E., Mesibov, G.B., & Hearsey, K. (1995). Structured teaching in the TEACCH system. In E. Schopler & G.B. Mesibov (Eds.), *Learning and cognition in autism* (pp. 243–268). New York: Plenum.

Schumm, J.S. & Vaughn, S. (1995). Meaningful professional development in accommodating students with disabilities. *Remedial and Special Education, 16*, 344–352.

Showers, B. (1990). Aiming for superior classroom instruction for all children: A comprehensive staff development model. *Remedial and Special Education, 11*, 35–39.

Sigafoos, J., Kerr, M., Roberts, D., & Couzens, D. (1994). Increasing opportunities for requesting in classrooms serving children with developmental disabilities. *Journal of Autism and Developmental Disorders, 24*, 631–645.

Smith, G. & Smith, D. (1985). A mainstreaming program that really works. *Journal of Learning Disabilities, 18*, 369–372.

Whelan, R.J. & Simpson, R.L. (1996). Preparation of personnel for students with emotional and behavioral disorders: Perspectives on a research foundation for future practice. *Behavioral Disorders, 22*, 49–54.

Index

Preschool services (*cont.*)
  Individualized Support Project (University
    of South Florida), 145–146
  LEAP program, 144–145
  legal foundations for, 142–143
  of May Institute, 144–145
  parental programs, 114
  Pivotal Response Model (University of
    California), 145–146
  of Princeton Child Development Institute,
    144–145
  schedules in, 148
  service provision models of, 143–144
  TEACCH approach. *See* Structured
    Teaching approach, in preschool
    programs
  university-affiliated, 143–146
  University of Colorado program, 144–145
  of Walden Preschool (Emory University),
    144–145
  Young Autism Project (University of
    California), 144–145
Princeton Child Development Institute,
  144–145
Program for Infants and Toddlers with
  Disabilities, 142–143
Prompts, as teaching technique
  in preschool programs, 149
  in social skills training, 94
Pronoun reversals, 57
Prosody, 59, 64
Psychoeducational Profile (PEP), 7, 9
Psychoeducational Profile (PEP)-Third
  Revision (PEP-3), 9
Psychoeducational Profile Revised (PEP-R), 4,
  147, 151
Psychology, developmental, 52
Public education, free appropriate (FAPE),
  142–143
Public Law 99–457 (Education of Handicapped
  Children Act), 142–143

Questioning, repetitive/persistent, 79, 82–83,
  183

Receptive understanding, in communication,
  59, 75
Rehabilitation Act Amendments of 1986,
  158
Reichler, Robert, 8, 106
Reinforcement, naturally occurring, use in
  social skills training, 94–95
Relaxation techniques, 170
Role playing, 95, 195
Rote memory skills, 65

Routines
  autistic individuals' attachment to, 26–27,
    54, 58
  Joint Action, 71
  in social interactions, 93
  in Structured Teaching, 43
  violation of, as communication stimulation
    technique, 71
Rutgers University, 143–144
Rutter, Michael, 10–11

Scaffolding, linguistic, 69, 72–73, 79
  in social skills training, 95–96
Scapegoating, 5
Schedules
  in adult services, 160
  in preschool programs, 148
  visual/pictorial, 41–43, 53–54
    in adult vocational programs, 166–167
    as response to persistent questioning,
      82
  use in transitions, 169
Schopler, Eric, 15–16, 33, 106
Scripts
  verbal, 71
  written, 70–71
Semantics, 59, 64
Sensory perception, effect on language
  development, 62
Sensory processing deficits, in people with
  autism spectrum disorders, 2–3, 26
Sequencing, autism-related deficits in, 24, 53,
  58
Sharing behavior, 92
Sign language, 36, 66
  in combination with oral language, 67
Social behavior deficits. *See* Social skills
  deficits
Social class, of parents of children with autism,
  109–110
Social-communications skills, preverbal,
  69–70
Social feedback, 93–94
Social phobia, in parents of children with
  autism, 111
Social reinforcement, 39
Social rules, violation of, 93
Social skills
  development of, 91–92
  influence of early experiences on, 142
  loss of, as autism spectrum disorders
    diagnostic criteria, 142
Social skills deficits
  in individuals with autism spectrum
    disorders, 3, 27–28, 91, 92–94